INTERMITTENT FASTING FOR WOMEN OVER 50

Accurate Guidelines to Start A Diet
To Improve Your Life

Table of Contents

Introduction

I f you've turned 50, then you probably know the joys of having to eat less and exercise more.

While there are a ton of lifestyle changes that you can make to look good and live longer, eating better is one of the most important ones. The value of a healthy diet cannot be overstated: it controls your weight, protects against disease, and even adds years to your life.

An emerging trend that could have major benefits for women over 50 who want to maintain their independence is the use of intermittent fasting. This involves going without food for a defined period each day (typically 16-24 hours) while drinking water or non-caloric beverages during this time frame.

The benefits of intermittent fasting have been mostly studied in men, but recent studies of women showed that eating regularly for 16 hours a day didn't mean that their health suffered.

Women are especially good at preserving lean body mass as they age, which is one of the reasons why they can survive without any regular food intake for months at a time. If your target is to lose weight, you need to eat regularly during the day and not overeat.

A 16-hour fast each day would work well for many women over 50 who want to improve their health and maintain their independence. As well as more energy, it will help you maintain or improve bone density and muscular strength, and stamina.

If you're going to use this method to improve or maintain your health, then you need to do so regularly. There is little benefit if you fast just once in a while, and it could actually be counter-productive.

The benefits of fasting also increase with duration: extending the time from 16 to 18 hours (18/6) has a greater effect than extending the time from 20 to 24 hours (24/1).

The longer you fast, the more weight loss benefits you get, but it also requires more self-discipline and patience. It also requires that you don't drink alcohol as it will stop your liver from burning fat for energy.

If you're going to try intermittent fasting, then do so because you want to have more control over your weight and better health.

The 16/8 method involves eating only within an 8-hour window each day. For example, if your last meal is at 3 pm then the next time you can eat is at 11 am the next day. You can have food whenever you want within this time window.

For most people, this means skipping one meal each day, but it could be two meals or more depending on how much food you eat and what time you like to eat. In fact, you can experiment to see which of the 8-hour windows works best for you. Ideally, it shouldn't be hard to stay within your window: in general, people eat a balanced diet that is rich in fiber and low in sugar and fat.

The main advantage of this method is that it can help you lose weight more easily than a traditional diet. For example, if you have a snack during your window then weight loss will be slower than if you were not hungry during this time.

We know that hunger can play a big part in how much we eat, but with intermittent fasting, hunger goes away completely until the next feeding window (typically 12 hours later). So it's important to not overeat and have small meals instead of large ones.

If you want to lose weight you should be eating a healthy diet that is low in sugar and fat while making sure your calorie intake is above maintenance. Having a snack during the time window will help you lose weight. The snacks can be something as simple as fruit, or it could be something like a nut butter sandwich on wholemeal bread (no added sugar).

If you're used to eating a high-sugar diet then intermittent fasting will take some getting used to, but if your goal is to eat better, then, this is an important change that might help.

The interesting thing about intermittent fasting is that it seems to overcome one of the limitations of the 16/8 method often used in weight loss studies. In these studies, people who went without food for longer than 14 hours didn't lose any more weight than those who fasted for 16 hours.

Going without food for 18 hours (18/6) has a better effect on losing weight, but most people need to eat a large meal at lunchtime. This is because they are usually hungry by the end of their fast and they can't wait until the next feeding window.

Another consideration is that you should not eat too close to bedtime as it can affect sleep quality. It is best to have a light snack in the afternoon and then eat your main meal in the evening.

Fasting for longer than 48 hours can be dangerous, so if you're going on long-term fasts (for example a ten-day fast) make sure you get some nutrients during this time. You would typically need to take sufficient nutrients to sustain yourself for at least one day after resting normally. You should also check with your doctor and do a blood test before embarking on any fasts of more than 48 hours as it may be medically required as part of a medication regime or diet.

CHAPTER 1:

What is Intermittent Fasting?

Intermittent fasting is a diet that consists of periods of fasting and periods of eating, usually 24 hours a day or more. It has been called the new Hollywood diet because many celebrities are following it, and it's being researched to see if and how it might help with weight loss.

The idea first came about in the 1930s when American medical doctor Dr. Ilia Petrovich teamed up with Dr. Albert Mattson to study whether a person who had food during 8 hours could live more healthfully than by just eating 2–3 meals per day. They learned that this idea was viable and in fact, a more efficient way to fuel the body.

The idea of intermittent fasting (IF) is not a new one. Ancient cultures around the world have practiced it for centuries. Many of those ancient cultures did not eat breakfast and used fasting to cleanse their bodies. They fasted every day for 1–3 weeks at a time, eating nothing but water or juices during those times.

This practice has continued along in many forms through the centuries: some people only fast once or twice a year for special occasions such as religious holidays, while others consider fasting as often as every other day to be part of their regular daily routine. Fasting has also been viewed as a way to lose weight.

The 16/8 diet, or the 8-hour diet, is one of these fasting diets. It requires people to fast every day for 16 hours of the day and eat only within an 8-hour window of time. Some people do not eat anything during their fasting period, while others can have fruits, tea, coffee, or water (but no solid food).

Why Would You Want to Fast?

Some proponents believe that when you fast you are allowing your body to focus on repair work without having to be burdened by digestion. Your cells get a chance to heal themselves and regenerate. You are also cleaner and healthier in general. Fasting also has been proven to lower cholesterol, blood pressure, and blood glucose levels.

Some people use fasting to prepare for a special occasion like a wedding feast or religious observance. While others do it when they want to get back into spiritual clean living, take a break from their usual eating habits, or go on vacation without the worry of prepared food that will spoil or be too expensive while away from home.

The 16/8 diet has long been advocated as an effective way to lose weight. It was featured on the 2010 cover of Shape magazine and drew attention for its ability to help women lose weight fast without serious health risks.

Anyone who's dieting knows that one of the major problems in weight loss is that hunger can overwhelm you by the time you get home from work and it's time to eat dinner. With the 16/8 plan, since you're not allowed to eat until 10 p.m., your hunger is diminished. You might even find yourself dropping a few pounds because your hunger is less intense and sharp.

Intermittent fasting is another version of a fasting plan that has been criticized as being too good to be true. Many people believe it is a fad diet that's too complicated or hard to maintain. Critics also claim the supposed weight loss is not real, just water weight.

Despite these objections, intermittent fasting has been embraced by many celebrities and other well-known people and is being studied by many scientists around the world. It is an interesting new way of eating that does not have the same risks as extreme dieting methods and a chance for people to eat healthier and lose weight if they try it.

CHAPTER 2:

Why Intermittent Fasting For Women Over 50?

Over the age of 50, it is increasingly difficult for a woman to lose weight and we are obsessed with those extra pounds that accumulate in areas where we do not want them to, such as hips and love handles. Intermittent fasting is an alternative to the usual diets, and can also become a way of life if you think of the countless benefits that calorie restriction brings to the body and mind.

The different types of intermittent fasting allow us to evaluate and choose the most suitable one for us, adapting it to our needs and lifestyle.

It is necessary to maintain a balanced and healthy diet, rich in vegetables and whole grains and that provides all the macronutrients needed by the body, as well as the right amount of fat (preferably vegetable) and avoid junk food, seasoned and too salty. All in all, however, you can eat anything, even taking a few whims from time to time.

Fasting has positive implications for the health of women over 50. Science has shown that reducing calorie intake prolongs life, because it acts on the metabolic function of longevity genes, reduces senile diseases, cancer, cardiovascular diseases, and neurodegenerative ones such as Alzheimer's and Parkinson's disease. Also, especially for women over 50, it has multiple benefits on mood, fights depression, contributes to the improvement of energy, libido, and concentration. And as if that weren't enough, it gives the skin a better look.

To start this type of "diet" you must first of all be in good health and any case, before starting, it is always better to consult your doctor. The female body is particularly sensitive to calorie restriction, because the hypothalamus, a gland in the brain responsible for the production of hormones, is stimulated. These hormones risk going haywire with a drastic reduction in calories or too long a fast. The advice is therefore to start gradually, perhaps introducing some vegetable snacks during fasting hours (fennel, lettuce, endive, radicchio).

As mentioned, in women, intermittent fasting works differently than in men. Sometimes it is more difficult for women to get results. Physiological and weight benefits are still possible but sometimes require a different approach. Besides, intermittent fasting on non-consecutive days is better able to keep those annoying hormones under control. Various scientific evidence shows that to achieve fat loss, fasting must be tailored to the sex.

For women, in particular, there are specific biological truths about fasting which, if you ignore them, will prevent you from achieving your goals of a better body and fitness. But there may be variations that allow you to overcome these problems. Fasting can prove to be a convenient and effective way to optimize your health and make you feel better, but only if it is done in a certain way: the way that is best for each of us.

Fasting, after all, represents the easiest and at the same time powerful detoxification and regeneration therapy that we can offer to cells and the whole organism. Putting certain functions at physiological rest does not mean that organs and tissues go on stand-by. On the contrary, thanks to the absence of a continuous metabolic commitment, they can dedicate themselves to something else, activating all those processes of self-repair, catabolism, excretion, and cell turnover that only in the absence of nutrients can take place at the highest levels.

Benefits and Differences on Women over 50

At the beginning, and especially the first few times, you don't realize what is happening inside, but it takes very little to feel the effects. Apart from the slight headache that can arise the first time, you usually feel more energetic, concentrated, and serene soon. Not only that, the perennial feeling of hunger turns into pleasant and constant satiety, which is maintained even after returning to normal nutrition.

Another effect of intermittent fasting, especially in overweight women, is to be able—without too much difficulty—to lose weight in the form of adipose tissue. Compared to a chronic low-calorie diet, an IF protocol can be a much more feasible and effective approach. There are many cases of women who, after trying it, learn to eat well even on feeding days. Obviously, it is not with DIY that lasting results are achieved, and I reiterate that any approach to FH should be planned with the whole dietary context in mind.

In normal-weight women, however, the effect on body composition is more unpredictable and controversial. Some expect to lose weight but are disappointed because the weight does not vary, and those who notice a better definition, especially in somebody areas.

In the first case, it is necessary to understand whether or not the desired weight loss was necessary at the outset, and especially if there are changes in body composition, which is much more important than weight itself. Weight loss, after all, should not be the first or only purpose of intermittent fasting. Some women may also experience morphological changes in their body, such as a thinning waist or a reduction in hip circumference, and this is certainly related to hormonal factors as well as changes in glucidic and insulin metabolism (better insulin sensitivity, less tendency to accumulate visceral fat). These different reactions allow us to make a very important reflection, which concerns the differences between one woman and another in terms of body composition and location of accumulations. For this reason, we must, first of all, make it clear which objectives we want to achieve and understand that every woman is different from the other.

Each woman is characterized by her constitutional type and endocrine profile, which determines a wide variability in terms of body composition, glucidic and lipid metabolism, and tendency to accumulate fat in localized areas. Some women with android conformation, for example, localize the largest reserves of adipose tissue at the abdominal level, while in gynoid women they more easily concentrate on thighs and buttocks.

It is clear, therefore, that it is useful to assess the suitability of each woman for intermittent fasting according to her body type.

CHAPTER 3:

How Intermittent Fasting Works

Intermittent fasting is the technique of scheduling your dishes for your body to obtain the most out of them. Rather than minimizing your calorie use by fifty percent, refuting yourself of all the foods you value, or diving right into a classy diet plan pattern, Intermittent fasting is an all-natural, logical, as well as healthy and balanced, and also balanced method of eating that advertises fat burning. There are tons of ways to approach Intermittent fasting.

It's defined as an eating pattern. This technique focuses on altering when you take in, instead of what you consume.

When you begin Intermittent fasting, you will be more than likely to maintain your calorie intake the same; nonetheless, in contrast to spreading your dishes throughout the day, you will undoubtedly eat more significant recipes throughout a much shorter amount of time. As opposed to consuming 3 to 4 meals a day, you might eat one big meal at 11 am, afterward an added large dish at 6 pm, without any dine-in between 11 am as well as 6 pm, as well as also after 6 pm, no meal up until 11 am is adhering to day. This is simply one strategy of recurring fasting, and likewise, others will be examined in this book in later stages.

Intermittent fasting is a technique used by whole lots of bodybuilders, specialist athletes, and also physical health and fitness masters to maintain their muscular tissue mass high and their body fat percent reduced. Recurring fasting can be done short-term or long-term, but the very best results originate from embracing this technique right into your everyday lifestyle.

The word "fasting" might stress the average person; Intermittent fasting does not associate with starving yourself. To comprehend the principles behind effective Intermittent fasting, we'll first review the body's digestion state: the fed state as well as the fasting state.

For 3 to 5 hours after consuming a meal, your body remains in what is described as the "fed state." Throughout the fed state, your insulin levels rise to soak up and digest your meal. When your insulin levels get high, it is exceptionally tough for your body to shed fat. Insulin is a hormone produced by the pancreatic to handle sugar degrees in the bloodstream. Its purpose is to manage insulin as technically a hormonal storage agent. When insulin degrees come to be so high, your body starts shedding your food for energy instead of your conserved fat. This is why boosted degrees of it protect against weight reduction.

After the 3 to 5 hrs are up, your body has finished refining the dish, and also you enter the post-absorptive state. The post-absorptive state lasts anywhere from 8 to 12 hours. When your body comes, hereafter the time room is the fasted state. As a result of the reality that your body has refined your food by this.

Factor, your insulin levels are reduced, making you kept fat extremely available for losing.

Persisting fasting allows your body to get to an innovative weight loss state that you would usually obtain with the average "3 meals daily" eating pattern. They are just altering the timing as well as the pattern of their food intake. It may take some time to get when you start an Intermittent Fasting program right into the swing of points. Merely obtain back if you slip up right into your Intermittent fasting pattern when you can.

Making a way of living adjustment entails a purposeful initiative, and also no one expects you to do it completely today. Intermittent fasting will take some getting used to if you are not in the practice of going long periods without eating. As long as you pick the right technique for you, continue to be focused, and also remain concentrated, you will unanimously grasp it quickly.

Unlike some of the other diet regimen strategies that you may embark on, the Intermittent fast will certainly work. When you listen to it, it is simple to obtain a bit terrified regarding fasting.

Recurring fasting is a little bit various than you might assume. If you finish up being on, your body will often go right into hunger mode, the rapid for as well lengthy.

You do not need to get as well concerned about exactly how this Intermittent quickly will work in the cravings mode. The Intermittent fast is efficient because you are not going too quick for as long that the body gets in right into this malnourishment setting as well as stops minimizing weight. Instead, it will make the rapid continue long enough that you will have the ability to accelerate the metabolic process.

With the Intermittent quick, you will discover that when you opt for a couple of hrs. without eating (usually no more than 2–4 hrs.), the body is not going to go right into a malnourishment setting. When complying with a recurring fasting plan, you require your body to melt more fat without placing it in any sort of extra job.

Here are a couple of fast pointers for success:

Mostly, it is essential not to expect to see outcomes from your new lifestyle promptly. Perhaps, you need to focus on devoting yourself to the process for a minimum of 30 days before you can start to evaluate the results correctly.

Second, it is imperative to remember that the excellent quality of the food you place into your body still matters as it will certainly merely take a few convenience food meals to reverse all of your tough work.

For excellent results, you will plan to consist of an in-light exercise routine during quick days along with a far more fundamental regimen for full-calorie days.

Recurring Fasting describes nutritional consumption patterns that include not consuming or continues limiting calories for a long-term period, Intermittent fasting (. There are various subgroups of regular fasting each with variance in the duration of the fast of individuals, some for hours, others for a day(s). This has finished up being an extremely liked subject in the clinical research area as a result of every one of the prospective advantages of fitness in addition to health that is being found.

The diet regimen you adhere to whilst Recurring fasting will be figured out by the results that you are looking for as well as where you are beginning with additionally, so take a look at it on your own and ask the question, what do I want from this?

If you are looking to lose a significant quantity of weight, then you are misting likely to have to take a look at your diet regimen plan extra closely, yet if you wish to shed a couple of pounds for the beach, then you could discover that a pair of weeks of Recurring fasting can do that for you.

There are many various ways you can do Recurring fasting. We just are most likely to consider the 24-hour fasting system in which is what I used to shed 27 pounds over a 2-month duration. You could really feel some cravings pains, but these will pass also, as you end up being even more familiar with Intermittent fasting you might find as I have that feeling of need no more existing you with a concern.

While fasting, it is suggested to drink a lot of water to avoid coffee, tea and dehydration are fine as long as you take a sprinkle of milk. If you are fretted that you are not getting adequate nutrients into your body, then you might consider a juice made from celery, lime, broccoli, and also ginger, which will taste fantastic and also get some sufficient nutrient fluid into your body. It would be best to stick to the coffee, water, and tea if you can handle it.

Whatever your diet strategy is whether it's healthy or not you should see weight reduction after three weeks of Intermittent fasting as well as do not be put off if you do not find much advancement at first, it's not a race, and also it is much far better to drop weight in a straight style over time as opposed to collision losing a couple of extra pounds which you will put right back on. After the initial month, you might want to have an appearance at your diet plan on non-fasting days and also remove high sugar foods and even any scrap that you might generally take in. I have discovered that intermittent fasting over the long-term tends to make me wish to consume healthier foods as an all-natural routine.

If you are practicing intermittent fasting for bodybuilding, then you may wish to consider having a look at your macro-nutrients and also working out just how much healthy protein as well as carbohydrate you call for to eat, this is a lot more complex, as well as you can uncover info about this on several websites which you will need to spend time examining for the very best results.

There are great deals advantages to recurring fasting, which you will view as you proceed, a few of these advantages include even more energy, much less bloating, a clearer mind, and a basic feeling of wellness. It's important not to succumb to any type of lure to binge eat after a fasting duration, as this will negate the influence obtained from the recurring fasting period.

In verdict simply by adhering to a two times a week 24-hour Intermittent fasting approach for a couple of weeks, you will slim down however if you can boost your diet plan on the days that you do not rapid then you will lose more weight and if you can remain with this system, then you will certainly keep the weight off without turning to any kind of fad diet regimen or diet plans that are difficult to stick to.

CHAPTER 4:

The Science of Intermittent Fasting

What Is Autophagy?

Autophagy is a process that happens within the human body that has been going on without our knowledge since the beginning of humans. It is only recently that people have begun to harness this process to achieve desired positive results through changes in their diet, such as Intermittent Fasting. We will look at this topic in-depth throughout this book, but here we will begin by looking at what exactly Autophagy is.

Autophagy, as a word, can be broken up into two individual parts. Each of these parts on its own is a separate Greek word—the word auto, which means self, and the word phagy, which means the practice of eating. Putting these together gives you the practice of self-eating, which is essentially what autophagy is. Now, this may sound a little intimidating, but it is a very natural process that our cells practice all the time without us being any the wiser. Autophagy is the body's way of cleaning itself out.

Essentially, the body has housekeepers that keep everything neat and tidy. Scientists who have been studying this for some time are not beginning to understand that there are ways to manipulate this process within your body to achieve things such as weight loss, improved health, reduction of disease symptoms, and so on. This is what we will spend the rest of the book looking at, but first, we will dive into the science of Autophagy a little more.

How Does Autophagy Work?

The process of autophagy involves small "hunter" particles that go around your body, looking for cells or cell components that are old and damaged. The hunter particles then take these cell components apart, getting rid of the damaged parts and saving the useful parts to make new cells later. These hunter cells can also use useful leftover parts to create energy for the body.

Autophagy has been found to happen in all organisms that are multi-cellular, like animals and plants, in addition to humans. While the study of these larger organisms and how autophagy works in their cells is lesser-known, more studies are being done on humans and how changes in diet can affect their body's autophagy.

The other function that autophagy serves is that it helps cells to carry out their death when it is time for them to die. There are times when cells are programmed to die because of several different factors. Sometimes these cells need assistance in their death, and autophagy can help them with this or can help to clean up after their death. The human body is all about life and death, and these processes are continually going on without our knowledge to keep us healthy and in good form.

As I mentioned, the process of autophagy has been going on inside of us for many, many years, since the beginning of humans. This process has been kept around inside of our bodies because of the multitude of benefits it can provide us with. It is also essential for the health of our bodies, as being able to get rid of waste and damaged parts that are no longer useful to us is essential to our health. If we were unable to get rid of damaged or broken cells, these damaged particles would build up and eventually make us sick. Our bodies are extremely efficient in everything that they do, and waste disposal is no different.

It is in more recent years that the study of autophagy has been focused more heavily on in terms of diet and disease research. These studies are still in their early stages as it has been only a few years shy of sixty years since autophagy was discovered. This process was discovered in a lab by testing what happened when small organisms went without food for some time. These organisms were observed very closely under a microscope, and it was found that their cells had this process of waste disposal and energy creation that was later named autophagy.

What Does Autophagy Do?

Autophagy is said to be the housekeeping function of the body. If you think of your body as your home, autophagy is the housekeeper that you hire to take care of all of the waste and the recycling functions of your cells.

One of the housekeeping duties includes removing cell parts that were built wrongly or at the wrong time. Sometimes cells make mistakes, and these mistakes can cause proteins or other cell parts to be formed in error. When this happens, we need something within the cell to get rid of these so that they do not take up space or get in the way of other processes within the cell. Further, sometimes useful parts of the cell will become damaged somehow and then will need to be removed to make way for a new part to take its place. These cell parts can include those that create DNA or those that create the proteins needed to make the DNA.

Another duty of autophagy is to protect the body from disease and pathogens. Pathogens are bacteria or viruses that can infect our cells and our bodies if they are not properly defended against. Autophagy works to kill the cells within our body that are infected by these pathogens to get rid of them before they can spread. In this way, autophagy plays a part in our immune system as it acts as a supplement to our immune cells whose sole function is to protect us from invasions by disease and infection.

Autophagy also functions to help the cells of the body to regulate themselves when there are stressors placed upon them. These stressors can be things like a lack of food for the cell or physical stresses placed on the cell. This regulation helps to maintain a standard cell environment despite factors that can change, like the availability of food. Autophagy can do things like break down cell parts for food to provide the cell with nutrients.

Similar to its role in the regulation of the cells, autophagy also helps with the development of a growing fetus inside of a woman's uterus. Autophagy occurs here to ensure that the embryo has enough nutrients and energy at all times for healthy development. In addition to this, it helps with growth in adults as well as there is a balance of building new parts and breaking down old ones involved in the growth of any organism.

Autophagy is more important than we may even realize, as it plays a large role in the survival of the living organisms it acts within. It does this by being especially sensitive to the levels of nutrients and energy within a cell. When the nutrient levels lower, autophagy breaks down cell parts, which creates nutrients and energy for the cell. If it weren't for this process, the cells would not be able to maintain their ideal functioning environment, and they may begin to make more mistakes and even lower their functioning abilities altogether. So much goes on inside of a cell that they need to be able to work effectively at all times. Autophagy makes this possible, which is what makes it such an essential function.

Using Intermittent Fasting to Induce Autophagy

Autophagy functions in the following way. When a decrease in nutrients is noticed within a cell, this decrease in nutrients acts as a signal for the cell to create small pockets within a membrane (a thin barrier layer) that are called autophagosomes. These small pockets (autophagosomes) move through the cell and find debris and damaged particles floating around within the cell. The small pockets then consume this debris by absorbing it into its inner space. The debris is then enclosed in the membrane (the thin barrier layer) and is moved to a place in the cell called the Lysosome. A lysosome is a part of a cell that acts as a center for degradation, breakdown, or disassembly. This part of the cell gets debris and damaged cell parts delivered to it by the autophagosomes. Once these damaged cell parts are delivered, the lysosomes then break them down. By breaking them down, these parts can be recycled and used for energy.

The most common way to induce autophagy in a person is by way of starvation. This is not to say that a person must starve themselves, but that they starve their cells of nutrition temporarily. This is why people turn to fast to induce autophagy. Low nutrition levels within the cells are the most common way that autophagy is triggered, as it is a process that creates energy within the cell. By knowing this, scientists have concluded that by inducing starvation within the cells, one can intentionally upregulate autophagy in one body. Intermittent Fasting involves periods of fasting, which then induces a state of starvation within the cells (simply meaning that there is no energy being consumed to use for energy) and so it induces autophagy in the cells to make energy.

Other Ways to Induce Autophagy

1. Starvation

The most common way to induce autophagy in a person is by way of starvation. Autophagy is triggered by a decrease in nutrients within a cell. As I mentioned above, this decrease in nutrients acts as a signal within the cell to begin the process of autophagy, which is exactly how Intermittent Fasting works.

2. Aerobic Exercise

One other way to activate autophagy is through exercise. Aerobic exercise has been shown through studies to increase autophagy in the cells of the muscles, the heart, the brain, lungs, and the liver.

3. Sleep

Sleep is very important for autophagy. If you have ever gone a few days without a proper, restful sleep, you know that you begin to feel a decline in your mental abilities rather quickly. This could be because of your brain's decreased autophagy functioning. The number of hours that you are in bed does not matter if the sleep is not good quality, though. Quality sleep for the right number of hours is what is needed to maintain good brain function and keep your brain's autophagy going.

4. Specific Foods

The consumption of specific foods has been shown to induce or promote autophagy. We will look at some examples of these foods later on in this book. The added benefit is that not only do they trigger autophagy in the cells of your body, these foods are also shown to have numerous other health benefits.

CHAPTER 5:

Guidelines To Start Your Intermittent Fasting

How to fast safely

Since there are so many risks involving intermittent fasting, it is important to take precautionary measures and opt for a safe road to achieving all its benefits. The following measures can help women of all ages, especially those over 50, to fast without causing any damage to their physical and mental health.

- **Choose the Right Method**

Intermittent fasting works differently for everyone, as the metabolic rates differ from one person to another. Just jumping into a routine, knowing only the benefits, can be dangerous. Women in this age group are advised to have a checkup first, calculate their body mass index and weight, look for any other health problems, and then choose a particular fasting method. Fasting every day might not help women who are diabetic. In this case, they must fast only for a short duration and with wider gaps to maintain their health. Start slow, then gradually increase the duration of the fast as the body adapts to the new regime.

- **Nutritional Needs**

Most women opt for intermittent fasting only to lose weight. In the weight loss struggle, they may turn a blind eye to their nutritional needs. Fasting does not mean depriving the body of what it needs to function properly. Therefore, meeting nutritional needs is imperative in this regard. Consume all the macro and micronutrients in your diet. Fibers, vitamins, minerals, phytonutrients are as important as proteins, carbohydrates, and fats for optimal brain and body function. The meal before and after the fast should be rich in quality, containing a wide range of nutrients.

• Eating is Essential

Do not go for a fasting method that would cause intense hunger pangs. Start with a short duration fast by adding a few hours to your normal gaps between the two meals. Eating is as essential as the fast itself. A complete abstention from food can result in malnutrition, so eat good and healthy food.

• Hydrate

When the body is in a fasting state, it goes into ketosis. Loss of water through increased urination is the direct outcome of ketosis. Dehydration can lead to electrolyte imbalance in the body. Therefore, it is very important to constantly hydrate yourself. During the fast, women can drink water, zero-calorie juices, and drinks to maintain the natural water levels of the body. Two to three liters of water consumption in a day are necessary when you are on intermittent fasting.

• Steadily Break the Fast

You may feel a predilection to eat everything at once when you break the fast. But this is an unhealthy act. Providing excessive nutrients to a fasted body at a time may lead to obesity and lethargy. It will reverse all the good effects of the fast. So, break your fast slowly by consuming small meals every half an hour during the FED state. Do not rely on a single meal; break it into several meals, ranging in flavors and ingredients to meet your nutritional needs. For instance, break your fast with a glass of smoothie, then leave a gap and follow with a protein-rich meal full of grains, fruits, and vegetables.

• No Overeating

Breaking the fast does not mean you can start stuffing your body with every edible item. Overeating is still harmful to a fasting regime. Remember, the goal of fasting is to restrict caloric consumption, and overeating does not help to achieve it. Therefore, avoid binge-eating after the fast and eat just enough to meet the body's basic needs of energy, vitamins, mineral, and fibers.

• Balanced Meals

A balanced meal contains high doses of protein and controlled amounts of fats along with smaller amounts of carbs, paired with traces of minerals, vitamins, and fibers. Whatever you eat before or after the fast, make sure to maintain this balance. For example, if you are cooking a delicious steak for your meal, then add some sautéed vegetables or whole grains, a drizzle of olive oil, some grated cheese, nuts, and seeds.

• Switch Between Time Periods

There is no fixed formula to fast! There are several methods to choose from, and a person can switch from one method to another, depending on the changes they are experiencing. As women over 50 are constantly going into hormonal and physical changes, they can turn to other methods of fasting if the method they are following isn't working for their health. Your fasting regime should only be health-centric; it doesn't have to be tied to a specific number of hours or days.

• Work Out

Most women over the age of 50 start considering themselves too old to exercise as they experience weakening of bones and lowering of the metabolism. But exercise is proved to be crucial in harnessing the benefits of a fast and healthy diet.

But it is recommended for women in their 50s not to over exhaust themselves during the fasting state. Only 10 to 15 minutes of light exercises are enough to keep you fit and active.

• **Monitor the Changes**

Without keeping track of the changes that your body experiences after fasting, you can't maintain a healthy routine. Women in their 50s should look out for any sign of discomfort or other symptoms during the fast which are considered harmful. Monitor the blood sugar levels, hunger levels, change in body weight, and improvement in health conditions to keep track of the progress.

How to break the fast? Tips & tricks to break your fast

The way a person breaks the fast is as important as the fast itself. No matter which of the above-mentioned methods of fasting a person chooses, without consuming a healthy meal with balanced nutrients, the real benefits of a fasting regime cannot be achieved. Remember, the main aim of intermittent fasting is weight loss and boosting the metabolic rate to fight against several health problems. If the fast is not paired with a healthy diet, it will not lead to desirable results. It is the case with many people who complain about the inefficiency of intermittent fasting. When people opt for the fasting regime, they focus solely on the fasting state, and once that stage is over, they believe all the work is done; however, that is far from reality. The FED state of the fasting regime is much more important and should be controlled with much care and proper planning.

When the body goes into a fasting state, it experiences several gradual changes. The glucose levels reduce gradually as the fast goes on. Initially, when we break the fast, the body reacts by storing energy in the form of fats more than usual to prevent any future deprivation.

And when the body receives more calories than its immediate energy needs it will store the excess, thus leading to obesity. Therefore, it is imperative to consume a healthy and proportionate meal to avoid calorie excess-accumulation.

Have you ever felt dull and lethargic right after breaking the fast? That is commonly observed by people who usually fast. It is not the fast that makes a person feel low; rather, it is the meal after the fast which causes it. That is why intermittent fasting requires a healthy diet. The following considerations must be kept in mind before breaking the fast.

1. Go Slow

The meal consumed between the two consecutive fasting periods should indeed be rich enough to meet the body's nutritional needs, but overconsumption should be avoided at a time. Every person has his own metabolic pace, and the body only utilizes a portion of the meal depending on the needs. As the excess is stored as fats, no one should consume more than the body can use. When you break the fast, go slow on the meal and gradually add meals to the FED state. After a long duration fast, there is not much time left to have multiple meals, so people try to have everything at once. There is no harm in eating one big meal, but the FED state should not start with this heavy meal.

Think of the FED state as a multi-course meal; the more the courses, the healthier it will be. Start with an appetizer to break the fast. Give your body some time to process those calories and gain the minimum required energy. Such appetizers do not have to be high-carb meals, but fresh and organic food should be consumed as stated above.

About 1 or 2 hours after the first appetizer, go for a more proper meal, which can be anything ranging from soups, stews, grilled steaks, seafood, satays, etc. This meal should be filled with a wide range of nutrients; you can always add a side dish like salads or dips, etc. When you are done with this meal, give your body a break for 4–5 hours until you will have the next meal, right before the fast. There can be two or three meals between the two consecutive fasting periods, depending on how long the fast lasts. Intake of juices and water must remain constant during this time.

2. Avoid Binge Eating

Binge eating is defined as uncontrolled consumption of food, and when a person breaks a fast, it may push him to binge eat all types of food just to satisfy the cravings. When you have low blood glucose levels, it leads to more cravings and vigorous eating. It is hard to resist for those who are already suffering from binge eating disorders.

Eric Stice, Kendra Davis, Nicole P. Miller, and C. Nathan Marti studied the relation between binge eating and fasting. The study was conducted on 496 participants who were put on the fasting regime. About 23 % of the participants showed a prominent sign of binge eating tendency and bulimia nervosa. The study concluded that people who fast can develop the tendency of binge eating more than people who are on other calorie restriction diet plans. Thus, people who fast need to fight against tendencies to binge eating. Breaking one single meal into multiple meals or adding more side dishes and snacks to the FED state of the fasting regime can help you resist the craving for excessive food consumption. Keep a constant intake of low or zero-calorie beverages all the time; this will prevent the urge to eat. Use fillers like leafy green vegetables and low-carb fruits to cope with food cravings. Remember, the whole fasting program is designed to restrict the daily or weekly caloric intake, and binge eating during the FED state can make this goal unachievable. So, while you restrict food during the fasting period, you must also avoid overconsumption when breaking the fast.

CHAPTER 6:

Differences Between Intermittent Fasting And "Fad Diets"

It is always easy to get caught up in the swirl of the latest fads and health crazes. While these have their merits, it's hard not to be skeptical when you see something like an all-chocolate diet or a carbohydrate-free lifestyle—especially if you know that it's only going to last for a week.

However, some diets are worth taking notice of intermittent fasting, for example.

Even though fad diets are usually short-lived, intermittent fasting is a diet that's been around for thousands of years. It was first used back in the 5th century BC as a method of weight loss and has even been featured in many ancient texts, such as The Art of Living by Epictetus: "Fasting is not a problem for the healthy man… It is rather something that even healthy people do on some days to clear up illnesses or to gain energy." However, before we delve into what intermittent fasting entails and how it can benefit you, we need to cover a few ground rules.

Firstly, not all diets last just a week. Intermittent fasting isn't even a diet in the sense that you are cutting out or changing your eating habits in any way. Instead, the only thing that you need to do is switch from eating your usual three meals per day to two per day. Now, instead of having breakfast, lunch, and dinner, you should have breakfast and dinner. It could be argued that this is still a diet because although the amount of food remains the same (you have just turned one of your meals into a smaller snack), you are consuming fewer calories for weight loss purposes.

Secondly, not all fad diets have little to no scientific evidence behind them. While the chocolate diet may be fun, there isn't any reputable evidence that it is healthy or works. On the other hand, intermittent fasting does have a lot of support and proof from various health studies. It was mentioned earlier that intermittent fasting has been used for thousands of years, but let's be honest - it's only in recent times that humans have started to live so long and can afford to worry about things like their waistline and cholesterol levels. One of the biggest health buzzwords in today's society is longevity: living as long as possible with the best possible quality of life. A prime example of this was the CALERIE-2 study that took place in 2010. This saw 215 people over the age of 25 participate in 6 months of calorie restriction, with one group cutting their calorie intake by a third and another group cut theirs by two-thirds.

You may be wondering why you would restrict your calories when eating is the most enjoyable thing in life! This kind of diet will indeed affect your mood and energy levels but scientists are constantly researching new ways to ensure that people can eat a lot and still reap the benefits of calorie restriction.

Scientists are also trying to understand the mechanisms behind calorie restriction. Studies have shown that by cutting down your calories, you limit your growth of any fat cells. Besides, this reduction in food intake leads to a higher level of antioxidants and lower levels of damaging free radicals which can affect your overall health and longevity dramatically. While there are many different types of intermittent fasting, the most common form is called 16/8so-called because you fast for 16 hours and have an 8-hour eating window (usually from noon until around 8 pm). This is when you would choose to eat and drink all three meals and snacks. This plan works out at about 600 calories per meal and a total of around 1,400 calories for the whole day. You should be aware, however, that this can lead to an overall calorie deficit of up to 1,600 calories per day—which isn't healthy and will make you lose weight regardless of the fact you are taking in a good amount of nutritious food.

This means that it is extremely important that you don't cut out certain types of foods—try to keep all meals as balanced as possible. For example, if you usually have a meal with carbohydrates (such as pasta), try instead to opt for complex carbs (like potatoes) or whole-grain carbs. This is because complex carbs have fewer calories per serving and usually provide more nutrition.

If you are feeling down or tired after the first week, remember to try and drink as much water as possible: your body is going through a tough time and needs all the nutrients it can get! Some people argue that it's not fair to call intermittent fasting a diet because you aren't cutting out any food groups. However, studies have shown that intermittent fasting can help improve your cognitive health and even be used as an effective treatment for certain neurological disorders. So, you can look at it as a way of improving your overall health and decreasing the risk of illness in the future.

Intermittent fasting has a lot of good things to say about itself. By simply restricting you're eating times, you're making it much easier for your body to have its energy needs met throughout the day. Unlike with more restrictive diets that can leave you feeling hungry and deprived, having this plan will allow you to skip straight to your meals and know that they are all coming at different times each day, so that will help with compliance too.

The other downside is the difficulty of removing yourself from when you want to fast. Many people find themselves in the situation where they have a dinner date and would like to fast that day. Or perhaps you love the idea of eating in on a special day but with a busy schedule of your own, you can't make it work.

However, many people find that fasting is very difficult if they are currently overweight or obese. In fact, around 80% of those who have issues with obesity report that their weight gain has been due to their inability to control their eating habits consistently. Water-soluble fibers found in legumes and lentils can become quite bulky, which makes them harder for your digestive system to break down. This can have negative effects on blood sugar and insulin levels, which would be problematic for someone trying to eat at their normal hours.

CHAPTER 7:

Macronutrients

What are Macros?

You have probably heard the term "macronutrients" before, or at least you've heard the term "macros." In many cases, you will hear people on the ketogenic diet talking about them because tracking them is a huge part of that regimen. Tracking your macros should be a huge part of just about any regimen, regardless of it being ketogenic or not.

Macronutrients are, quite simply, the nutritional compounds or elements that you're putting into your body when you eat. The most common ones to watch are protein, carbohydrates, and fats. The reason for looking at these is to make sure that you're keeping things in an adequate balance in your diet. If you're eating mostly fat without eating enough protein or enough carbohydrates, your body will react differently. If you know you need to be eating a certain amount of protein each day, then you will keep a keener eye out for the things that have more of it like chicken breasts, or other lean meats, as they will add protein without adding considerable fat.

In most cases, there aren't rigid numbers you need to stick to for each of these while doing intermittent fasting. It is important, however, that you're not taking on foods that are mostly carbs or fat while you're dieting, right? If you want to make sure that your body is going to get the most out of the things, you're eating without feeling sluggish or putting on excess weight, you're not going to be eating things that are primarily carbohydrates either.

Carbohydrates

Your body will primarily use carbs as its means of fuel and most typical diets will dictate that you make up your diet with about 45%-65% carbs. Your body will use carbohydrates as fuel for just about every internal process it has. Your body can very easily break down carbohydrates, making it a convenient fuel source when taken on in the right amounts. There are some doctor-recommended programs for those who need to reduce their weight that require that this percentage be drastically reduced, but that's not typical.

Carbohydrates, when they break down, are converted into glucose, which is the real raw fuel your body can use to keep moving. Glucose is absorbed into the cells of your body, fueling each one's processes. When your body ends up with an excess of glucose, it gets converted once more into something else called glycogen which is converted into the fat stores your body keeps for future use. This is sort of an evolutionary holdover that allows you to get through periods of starvation, as the food was far scarcer than it is today. However, most of us are in no position to starve and those fat stores stick around doing no good for anyone until we work them off.

One of the things to bear in mind when you're evaluating whether or not to cut carbohydrates is that there is no one type of carbohydrate and that deciding "carbs are bad," is not as black and white or correct as it might seem. There are simple carbohydrates and there are complex carbohydrates.

The labels "simple" and "complex" refer to the length of the molecule itself, which is not something you'll be able to tell just by looking at the food. You will, however, be able to know it by whether or not the food is processed. Simple carbohydrates that take your body almost no time to burn through and your body will typically be left with more glycogen at the end of that process. Complex carbohydrates take a longer time to break down in the body and give your body more fuel in the time it takes to break them down.

Simple carbohydrates are mostly sugars, so you'll find those in candies, sodas, juices, and things like that. Complex carbohydrates are in things like bananas, legumes, and whole grains.

There is no black and white answer about whether simple or complex carbs are better or worse for you, but you will generally find that complex carbs are much better for lasting power. You will, however, find that if you avoid processed foods, you will feel better and get the most out of the carbs that you do eat!

Protein

Proteins are used to build muscle and repair the body to keep it going from day to day. That's why you need more protein if you decide to start working out and exercising more. Your body needs to recuperate and repair and protein is the ideal helper for that process. It's recommended that about 20%-35% of your daily intake is made up of proteins. The protein that you take on allows your body to restore cells, to grow, to grow your hair and nails, to repair and refresh your skin, and all that very essential stuff! This doesn't mean that eating 100% protein will help your body regenerate like a comic book character, but it does mean that it's quite important to ensure that you're getting enough protein!

You get essential amino acids from the foods that you eat, and those will often come from the animal proteins that you eat. There are 20 amino acids and nine of those aren't produced in our bodies. They're classified as essential because we need to get them from the foods that we eat, namely the animal proteins. If you're a vegetarian, you can get them from sources of plant-based protein.

Fat

Over the decades, you've likely watched the stigma and public opinion surrounding fats evolve. For a while, every diet food was fat-free, then there was the Atkins craze and food couldn't have enough fat in it to satisfy shoppers and dieters, and it's been an ever-evolving cycle ever since. Without getting too confusing about the truth of fats, here is the long and short of it. Fats should take up about 10%-35% of your daily intake. Of those fats, you want to make sure that as many as possible are "good fats."

This means you want fats from lean protein sources, fats that contain Omega-3 fatty acids, Omega-6 fatty acids, and which don't come from overly processed foods. These come from things like fish, walnuts, eggs, and vegetable oils. When foods naturally have fat in them without any help from processes like homogenization or emulsification, you will generally find the fats to be good. The fats in dairy are helpful to the body in moderation, and if you aren't lactose intolerant.

You can also look for these things:

Saturated Fats: These come from meat, dairy, and other animal byproducts.

Unsaturated Fats: These are the plant-based fats that come from veggies, nuts, and the like.

Trans Fats: These types of fats are generally only produced in the commercial production and processing of foods like fast foods, snack foods, and butter substitutes that aren't plant-based.

Trans fats should be avoided for the most part, if not entirely, as those are fats your body can't particularly use and which don't contribute to healthy heart function.

What Should My Macros be During Intermittent Fasting?

There is no set amount of each macro that you should be taking on each day when you're doing intermittent fasting. You will find that you generally want to keep to the percentages outlined above for your macros. That means that you should be eating enough to fill yourself up without going overboard. In many cases, you will lose weight on intermittent fasting because you won't eat as much as you otherwise would.

Those macros once again are:

Carbs: 45% to 65%

Protein: 20% to 35%

Fats: 10% to 35%

If you can make sure your macros are just about in this range, then you will often find that you are feeling your best and that you are doing quite well. If you need the help of a calorie-tracking app, you might find that you're more able to stay on top of your intake and that you're able to feel fuller for longer without overdoing it.

It's not completely necessary to watch your calories to do intermittent fasting and to feel the benefits that it has to offer, but it can help you to keep on track and to keep yourself from doing things you wish you hadn't.

Unfortunately, many of us are not familiar with serving sizes and how many of the things we're supposed to be eating in a sitting. Many of us have taken out cues from the restaurants around us and, the horrible truth is that the average restaurant will serve you 2–3 times as much as you're supposed to be eating in one sitting!

If you have found yourself wondering why you're not losing weight when you think you've been eating everything in moderation, it could be worth it to track your calorie and food intake on one of those apps to see what you're taking in.

CHAPTER 8:

Health and Esthetic Benefits of Intermittent Fasting

Lifestyle Benefits

When compared to other diets, the simplicity of intermittent fasting makes it perhaps the easiest eating protocol through which to experience significant health benefits. Often, the complexity of some eating plans causes people to fail at the first hurdle because as much as they think they understand what they should be doing, they don't. This results in people going to punishing extremes to fulfill what they think they are supposed to be doing and ending up with very disappointing results. Intermittent fasting couldn't be simpler—now you eat and now you don't. Often, special diets can be extremely expensive to follow. You have to purchase special ingredients and eat food that you ordinarily wouldn't. Intermittent fasting is different in that regard too. It costs you absolutely nothing to practice intermittent fasting, and other than a caloric reduction in the case of weight loss and eating as healthy as possible, there is no dictation as to what to eat.

Intermittent fasting is flexible, so it allows you gaps in between to eat the things you enjoy. What is life without an occasional dessert, some chocolate, or pizza? With intermittent fasting, you can have those treats and not feel guilty because when you fast, your body will be burning that treat off. Of course, that is not to say that in every eating window you can binge on every fast food known to mankind. You will still need to eat a healthy diet; you just won't be weighing food and calculating its calorie content all the time.

If you have found an eating plan that you enjoy such as Keto, Paleo, or the like, you can incorporate that with intermittent fasting. There are no other plans available where you can combine two and get even better results. Intermittent fasting is a fantastic addition to other eating plans and does not detract from any other diets (Fung, 2020).

For women over 50, the adjustment to menopause can mean a temporary lifestyle change. In severe situations, menopause can result in difficulties in relationships with partners and loved ones. Intermittent fasting can help make a big difference in these challenges, and this can be life-changing.

Health Benefits

Cardiovascular health should be a strong focus for people of all ages but even more so for women over 50. The most significant cause of death for women over 50 today is cardiovascular disease. This umbrella term describes all diseases of the heart or the arteries leading to and from the heart. This could include blockages, damage, and deformities in the structure. Several risk factors contribute to the occurrence of cardiovascular disease including smoking, physical inactivity, genetics, and diet. The latter, however, is the largest controllable contributor to heart disease.

The most impactful factor where diet is concerned is the types of protein sources that are eaten as well as the types of fats that are consumed. Plant proteins such as beans and legumes have been proven to be a healthier source of protein than animal proteins in general.

Where animal protein is concerned, the leaner the source, the better, and poultry, and fish are always healthier options than red meat. The fat component of red meat is another problem where heart disease is concerned, as are other sources of fat such as cooking oils and spreads used for bread. Saturated fats are the types of fats we want to avoid in our diet, and these include animal fat, lard, and tropical oils such as palm oil. Unsaturated fats in small quantities are healthier. Examples of unsaturated fats include avocados, nuts, olive oil, and vegetable oils. When we eat foods over what our body can burn, the leftover food forms triglycerides that, at high levels, contribute to the occurrence of cardiovascular disease. When we fast, our body burns triglycerides for energy thereby reducing the levels in our blood and, in turn, reducing our risk of cardiovascular disease.

This decrease in insulin results in less food being stored as fat. In animal trials, intermittent fasting has been shown to prevent and reverse Type 2 Diabetes. Another thing that happens when insulin levels decrease is that the FOXO transcription factors, which are known to positively impact metabolism, become more active in the body. This process is also linked to improved longevity and healthy aging.

Another noncommunicable disease that seems to be impacted by intermittent fasting is cancer. Growth Factor 1 (GF1) is a hormone very similar in nature to insulin, and the presence of this hormone is known to be a marker for cancer development. Levels of GF1 are reduced during intermittent fasting. Women over 50 are twice as likely to develop breast cancer, for instance, and risk factors for other common cancers are also thought to increase when women start to experience the hormonal changes of menopause. Intermittent fasting is, therefore, an excellent preventative measure for the occurrence of cancer in women over 50.

The increased cell resilience seen in people who regularly fast has been linked to a stronger immune system as well as a general faster recovery from illness. The process of building cell resilience through fasting is similar to exercising muscles. The more you undertake regular exercise with periods of rest in between, the stronger your muscles become.

The autophagy process that is triggered by intermittent fasting has been shown to help reduce inflammation in the body as well as oxidative stress, which is primarily responsible for cell damage in the body. Inflammation in various parts of the body is present as a precursor to the diagnosis of many different non-communicable diseases. The diagnosis of non-communicable diseases is far more common in women over 50 than any other age group. It is, therefore, vital for women in this age group to make use of intermittent fasting and autophagy as an additional preventative measure against the development of noncommunicable diseases.

The Circadian Cycle is the name given to the rhythm created in our body by light and dark (day and night). This natural rhythm controls our need to sleep and eat and has a major impact on our metabolism, cognitive function, and emotional health. It is our internal clock, and when disrupted, it can have devastating effects on our bodies. Intermittent fasting has been shown to help regulate the Circadian Cycle and, if it is out of the loop, reset it back to its natural function.

From an evolutionary perspective, our bodies are designed to eat during the day and not to eat at night. This, of course, is the reverse in certain nocturnal mammals who have evolved to reverse that Circadian Cycle due to the availability of prey at night. As modern humans, we have disrupted our Circadian Cycle by not going to sleep when the sun goes down and also continuing to eat well into the night. This impacts our metabolism and our sleeping patterns, resulting in weight gain and sleep disorders such as insomnia. By using intermittent fasting to reset our internal clock to its evolutionary default, we can encourage weight loss by optimizing our metabolism and have a more restful sleep.

In women over 50, this is particularly beneficial. As we age, sleep disorders become more common. We feel tired earlier, experience disturbed sleep, and generally find that we are unable to sleep for as many hours as we once could. This sleep disruption, of course, has a major impact on our health both physically and mentally. The reason for this change in sleep is due to the reduced levels of Human Growth Hormone (HGH) in our bodies as we age. As we now know, intermittent fasting helps to increase the levels of HGH in our body, thus allowing us to regain a more regular sleeping pattern.

If you eat too long before you go to bed, you may experience hunger pangs while you sleep that disrupt your sleep. If you eat too large a meal before going to sleep, your body will still be diverting additional blood flow to your stomach to digest its contents, and that will also disrupt your sleep. The importance of a good sleeping pattern cannot be understated as poor sleeping patterns have even been shown to increase the likelihood of the occurrence of certain cancers.

Intermittent fasting has also been shown to improve the regulation of genes that promote liver health and also in the balance of gut bacteria. Gut bacteria play a role in our immune system, and it is vital to keep these gut guests in good shape to optimize your body's defense systems (Kresser, 2019).

Cognitive Functioning Benefits

As you move into your 50s, there are several different effects on your brain health and, as a result, your cognitive functioning. Brain shrinkage automatically occurs as we age, and although it is not something we can avoid, it is certainly something that we can delay and slow down. From a fasting perspective, the process of autophagy, which speeds up during fasting, can help to consume damaged brain cells and use that cellular material to produce new brain cells. This process can help to alleviate the natural brain shrinkage process.

The release of ketones during the burning of fat which occurs during fasting is also highly beneficial to brain health. The enhanced level of ketones helps to protect the brain from the development of epileptic seizures, Alzheimer's Disease, and other neurodegenerative diseases. Of course, as we age, we are also more likely to develop neurodegenerative diseases. Diseases like Alzheimer's and other forms of dementia do have a wide range of risk factors including genetics and smoking. Fasting to enhance autophagy and ketone production is one way that we put up a line of defense against these diseases.

Intermittent fasting can also help to improve neuroplasticity, which is the brain's natural capability to build new neural pathways. This is imperative in learning as well as in the breaking of habits. When we break bad habits, we work to remove the brain's reliance on a commonly used neural pathway and promote the use of a new pathway. Studies in people with brain injuries have shown that intermittent fasting speeds up healing.

CHAPTER 9:

Risk and Disadvantages of Intermittent Fasting For Women Over 50

Risks of Intermittent Fasting

The risks of intermittent fasting are varied. If people fast when they shouldn't, then the risks of intermittent fasting can be quite severe. However, for most people, intermittent fasting isn't very risky. The risks you'll run into are bingeing, malnutrition, and difficulty with maintaining the fast. We've talked about bingeing quite extensively, so we're not going to discuss it much more. Suffice it to say, bingeing while you fast risks any of the benefits from fasting you might originally have. A bigger risk is malnutrition.

Malnutrition sounds alarming, but for the most part, you can prevent this by having well-balanced meals during your eating windows. The risk of malnutrition comes especially during the kinds of fast which include a very-low-calorie restriction on fasting days. Fasts like this are 5/2 fasts and alternate-day fasting. If you're not eating the right nutrition throughout your week, the reduction in calories plus the poor nutrition can result in some of your dietary needs not being met. This could result in more weight loss, but also more muscle loss and other issues. To prevent this risk, you can ensure that your meals are nutritious and well-balanced. Have a variety of fruits and vegetables, try different meats and seafood, and include grains unless you're following a specific diet like the keto diet.

Associated with malnutrition is dehydration. We get a lot of our daily water intake from the food we eat. But if you're eating a reduced amount of food during your day, or no food during your day, you're going to need to drink a lot more water than you normally do. If you're not keeping track of your hydration levels, you can drink too little. To combat this risk, ensure that you're drinking enough by keeping a hydration journal. You could also track it in an app. Set up reminders to drink water and check your urine color. Light-colored urine means good hydration, so check often despite how disgusting it might be to you.

Because fasting can be difficult to start, this can be one of the risks associated with it. You're going to feel hungry during the first couple of weeks of following your fasting schedule. You may even feel uncomfortable, with mood swings, different bowel movements, and sleep disruptions. All of this can lead to you struggling with starting the fasts. They can also lead you to ignore greater warning signs that you shouldn't fast. These signs include changed heart rate, feelings of weakness, and extreme fatigue. These feelings shouldn't be ignored during the start. If you feel severely uncomfortable when you start your fast, you should stop and speak with your doctor.

Disadvantages of Intermittent Fasting

Unfortunately, intermittent fasting has cons too, especially for females. Studies show that before trying intermittent fasting, you should always contact your physician. The following are the disadvantages associated with intermittent fasting:

It is not risk-free: Intermittent fasting is not advisable to people who are at higher health risks such as those over sixty-five years. People under medical conditions, high fat needs, the diabetic, the underweight, the underage, pregnant, and those breastfeeding cannot undertake intermittent fasting.

You will be hungry: During intermittent fasting, you might have a grumbling stomach, especially if you have correctly been observing the correct dietary plans. You should avoid looking at, smelling, or even thinking about food while fasting since these triggers the releasing o gastric acids in your stomach, which then makes you hungry. Engage in some other activities but if you wish to fill your water, drink herbal tea or other drinks free from calories. You may note increased food intake in the non-eating days where you are not limited to any calorie intakes. Intermittent fasting triggers binge food consumption. There could also be cases of cravings, especially after increased levels of cortisol hormone.

Dehydration: Lack of eating may make you forget to take water. You might fail to take note of the thirst cues when fasting.

Fatigue: Intermittent fasting makes you feel tired, especially if you are trying it for the first time. Your body tends to run short of energy and disrupts your sleep patterns, and this comes along with a feeling of being tired.

Irritability: Since intermittent fasting helps in mood regulation, it can as well regulate your appetite. It leads to being depressed and upset.

Intermittent fasting long-term consequences are not known: Since no one knows whether after losing weight, you will maintain the same for some years, studies claim that no relevant evidence to support the extent of intermittent fasting. You are therefore always advised to talk to your doctor for sound advice on how you should practice intermittent fasting.

You should:

Ensure that your body is fit for fasting. It is by making sure that you are not pregnant, not under any medication, no health complications, not underage, or even diabetic. If you cannot fast, then you can always change to cleaner eating habits such as eating natural foods and eliminate any sugar, rich, or fatty foods from your diet.

Before starting intermittent fasting, you should always try and consult your doctor. Your doctor will give updates about your health concerns and advise whether the step is necessary or not.

Try and make intermittent fasting fit into your lifestyle. You should never fast during the times you are stressed or under excess exertion. It is advisable if you are a newbie in intermittent fasting to try the 5/2 way of fasting whereby you can fast on the first day of the week, then on Thursdays so that you can prepare to take your favorite meals over the weekend.

Before you start intermittent fasting, do not gorge yourself with a "last supper" but you should instead take healthy meals, lean proteins, and vegetables. Fruits have natural sugar and including them in your meal could mean a lot. A little amount of starch could make the meal complete, as well. A meal that has all these nutrients will make your body survive the fasting period.

Prepare your household, body, and thoughts before starting intermittent fasting. It means that you should have enough rest and get prepared emotionally. Think about your aim and how to achieve it. Make sure that you hide or keep out of reach any foods that could tempt you during your fasting period.

Stop pretending to be a hero, even when your body is weak. Do not push your body too hard in the name of fasting. There are some of the symptoms that should be of great concern during your fasting time. You should take note of heart shudders, light-headedness, and general feebleness. It requires the use of common sense because you cannot force your body to do what it cannot.

Do not engage in tough exercises; do light ones. Engage in massages as they help have even blood flow in the body parts full of calories, thus reducing cortisol. Do not burn the muscles for energy while fasting.

Always take your vitamins depending on the method of fasting you choose. That acts as a supplement, especially if in liquid form as it eases the process of digestion. They help compensate for the vitamins lost while fasting.

Never forget to take a lot of water every fasting day. Your t
alert you if it is not light in color. If not so, drink desirabl
water for proper hydration.

Since you are fasting, it is an obstacle to associating with your friends
who are having fun; eating chocolates, and drinking wine since you will
get tempted to take some. You can indulge in other ways of having fun
with your friends. You can pay a visit to the nearest mall, window-
shop new clothes or electronics. Avoid grocery stores and any dinner
dates. Clear any mouth-watering photos from your gallery.

Avoid getting stressed since stress increases the levels of cortisol,
which is responsible for fat storage and muscle breakdown. You can
practice yoga, meditating, or having deep breaths. Your body needs
enough energy to last you during the fasting period, and so these
exercises should be light and not vigorous.

To avoid freaking out, you can always invite your friends to
accompany you in doing intermittent fasting. The idea of creating
your fasting thread or checking online for any other people doing
intermittent fasting can help you master your progress. That is the time
that you should focus on mentally cleaning your closet and reflecting
on what you are doing.

Avoid "Victory Binging." Many people indulge themselves after the
fasting period. You should take in a healthy meal and avoid foods that
cannot get digested easily. You should take in foods rich in fiber and if
you are alcoholic, remember to take care when resuming.

CHAPTER 10:

Intermittent Fasting Types for Women

The 16/8 Method

The 16/8 method of fasting, also known as the Leangains protocol, is the most popular type of intermittent fasting. It was originally developed by Martin Berkhan, a nutritional expert and personal trainer who was looking for a way to help his clients build muscle without accumulating fat. When following the 16/8 method, you schedule a sixteen-hour fasting window and an eight-hour feeding window each day. For example, you may choose a fasting window between 7 p.m. and 11 a.m., which means the feeding window, would fall between 11 a.m. and 7 p.m.

There are no hard rules about the times you must eat, but once you decide on a schedule, you'll want to stick to it every day. If you don't have a consistent feeding window, it can throw your hormones out of whack and make it even harder to stick to the program because you'll experience more hunger and may not notice any of the positive health benefits. There are also no restrictions on the number of meals you eat: you can fit breakfast, lunch, dinner, and even some snacks into the eight-hour eating window. Of course, if weight loss is one of your goals, you'll want to be more mindful of your calorie intake.

Research shows that women over 50 years may do better with a fourteen or fifteen-hour fasting window and a nine or ten-hour eating window. If you are a woman and you want to follow the 16/8 method, start with a fourteen-hour fast and see how you feel. Easing into it will give your hormones time to adjust and will make any negative side effects, like changes in or loss of energy, less likely.

During your fasting window, you are allowed to drink water, coffee, and other non-caloric beverages, such as tea or seltzer; however, pay attention to your caffeine intake and be careful not to overdo it. While sipping beverages during your fasting window can help stave off hunger, too much caffeine can leave you anxious, jittery, and dehydrated, especially when your stomach is empty.

Caffeine also puts stress on your adrenals, so while your body is adjusting to the added stress of fasting, it's best to keep your coffee intake minimal. One of the major benefits of this method of intermittent fasting is that it's fairly easy to incorporate into your schedule. Since you'll be sleeping for around eight hours of your fast, you only have to skip food for a small portion of your waking hours. Most people can successfully pull off the 16/8 method by not eating after dinner and then skipping breakfast or eating it late in the morning.

The 5/2 Diet Method

The 5/2 intermittent fasting is another popular method of fasting that's followed by many people and involves an intake of 25% of your calorie needs. It's referred to as 5/2 since one is required to eat normally during the five days of the week and then restrict calories to between 500 and 600 per day for the two days. The 5/2 diet method is normally considered as an eating pattern and not a diet, and there are no specifics on the foods that can be eaten. Focus is instead on when the foods should be eaten. Since the intake of calories is reduced, you are, therefore more likely to lose weight.

To get started with this method of fasting, you can choose the two days within the week that you can reduce the intake of calories to 500. Ensure that there is one day of fasting in between the days you have chosen. You can fast on Monday, and Thursdays, as you take 2 to 3 small meals then resume your normal eating on the remaining days. Eating normally doesn't necessarily mean that you just eat anything; if you decide to binge on junk food, then you should be aware of the fact that you might not attain your goal.

The 5/2 diet is much easier to follow than the traditional diets that restrict calorie intake. This method can effectively lead to weight loss if undertaken well; however, the hunger that one gets to experience can be limiting for some. The limitation in calorie intake with 500 calories for women and 600 hundred for men for the two fasting days may help with improving brain functioning, amongst other benefits. This method of fasting also helps in repairing body cells which are likely to contribute to various health conditions.

When following this method of fasting; you don't have to go for a day without taking food; all you have to do is to ensure that at least the intake of calories for two days within the week is restricted to 500 for women and 600 for men. The limit in calories on the fasting days enables you to eat small quantities of food on specific days. You can choose whichever food you want to eat under this method as long as the intake of calories is limited to the required amount. To keep away hunger pangs, you can go for foods that are filling and those that don't have a lot of calories so that you can stay full for longer periods. Foods like leafy green vegetables and smaller portions of lean meat can be great if taken in the right quantities. Soups are also great and filling as well and remember to avoid consumption of processed carbohydrates such as bread or pasta.

The Eat-Stop-Eat Method

This method of fasting is also known as the 24 hours fast, and it's based on the understanding that our bodies are meant to be in a constant cycle of fasting and feeding. So when you consume a large amount of food, then the body gets to store fat that can be burned later whenever there is an inadequate supply of food. By engaging in regular yet short periods of fasting, then provides one with the simplest way of losing weight in a way that doesn't affect the metabolic rate. Fasting for 24 hours once a week or even twice a week is capable of producing results that are similar to one on very strict dieting. You, however, don't have to go for an entire day without eating if you follow the required guidelines.

The eat-stop-eat method can be practiced by eating normally until 6 pm in one day then fasting until 6 pm the following day. This method of fasting makes it possible for one to enjoy the benefits of fasting without having to stop eating for a whole day. To engage in fasting easily, you can think of fasting as if you are breaking from the normal eating routine. Remember to avoid any temptation to overeat once you complete the fast as engaging in excess eating may neutralize the benefits that come with practicing the fast. While on this method of fasting, you can also engage in resistance exercises as that helps in maintaining the muscle tissue.

You can adjust your training and exercises regarding intensity, frequency, and volume of training. You can also consider adding additional exercises, such as engaging in yoga, aerobics, or cycling. The eat-stop-eat fasting method is quite basic and easy to follow. You can decide to do the fasting once or twice a week but the fast should be for 24 hours. You can start at any time that you are comfortable with provided you maintain the fast to 24 hours. Break the fast with a normal meal and never try to compensate for the lost calories. Remember to also engage in exercises as you engage in fasting.

The Alternate Days Fasting

This is one of the extensively studied forms of short-term fasting, and just as the name implies, it entails fasting for some days each week and eating normally as you would. You can decide to fast on Monday, eat normally on Tuesday then fast again on Wednesday, and continue in the same manner. Alternate-days-fasting is a very flexible way of fasting, and you can plan your week effectively. The biggest challenge with this method is that it's not as effective when it comes to burning fat as a source of energy, getting the body into ketosis then highly depends on the quality of foods that one gets to eat when on the diet.

To practice this method with successful results, you can dedicate the first 24 hours to taking water and less than 500 calories. You can either take the calories in one meal or spread them all through the day. You can then eat whatever you want in the following 24 hours; however, you should emphasize taking a low-carb high-fat diet so that you are not thrown ketosis in the process. A high-fat diet is also satisfying, so you are likely to be filled for longer periods. If you are fasting for a day then eating the following day, then you should restrict whatever you are eating to half of the time.

On the days you are fasting, you can take beverages that are free of calories. The alternated-days-fasting is demanding, and you should be ready to follow through with the diet daily as required if you are to realize the benefits. Various studies show that most people find alternate-day fasting much easier to follow through with than the traditional everyday way of restricting calories. The intake of 500 calories on the fasting days makes the method to be sustainable than having full fasts on the fasting days. Alternate day fasting is quite effective for weight loss, and the fact that it's much easier to follow through with makes it quite ideal. The effects of alternate-day fasting on hunger are inconsistent with some studies showing that hunger tends to go down on the fasting days and others state that feelings of hunger remain. Modified alternate-days-fasting where you take 500 calories on fasting days is quite tolerable. It also causes favorable changes.

Crescendo Method

Crescendo fasting and Intermittent fasting way of life moves toward that have helped numerous individuals accomplish their wellbeing objectives. Fasting is an old mending system that has been utilized since the start of known history. Intermittent fasting is a type of fasting where somebody is fasting 12 to 16 hours or more every day. During this fasting window, you may not be expending anything aside from water or maybe homegrown tea. During the remainder of the day, you would eat a typical, solid eating regimen.

Intermittent fasting can have mind-blowing benefits, including lower aggravation, weight reduction, fat consumption, improved vitality, better processing, and improved association with nourishment, better mental and profound wellbeing, and a lower danger of ceaseless malady.

Be that as it may, male and female bodies unexpectedly respond to fasting. Women may confront expanded difficulties when fasting, including hormonal issues, insulin opposition, and affectability to calorie limitation. Notwithstanding, women can even now profit from Intermittent fasting, however, they may need to alter their methodology. Crescendo Fasting and Cycle Fasting might be incredible Intermittent fasting systems for some women.

We should jump into finding out about the advantages of Intermittent fasting, the contrasts among people more than 50 with regards to fasting, and indications of insulin obstruction and hypoglycemia. You will realize why I prescribe a straightforward fast and an early lunch fast to begin and afterward how to move onto Crescendo Fasting and Cycle Fast securely and adequately. I will likewise go through more than 7 techniques to improve your fasting experience.

CHAPTER 11:

How to Plan Intermittent Fasting

O nce you have established the type of intermittent fasting plan that best suits you, you can finally put the plan into action. There is no time like the present and it is wise to begin fasting as soon as you can, giving you less time to procrastinate about all the when, what, and ifs.

Setting up a basic plan of action is simple when it comes to fasting. Our pantries and refrigerators also do not need to be overpopulated with rare and expensive ingredients. Fasting is simple and it can be done, more than likely, with the items you already have stored in your kitchen cupboards. Creating a plan of action is the sure-fire way in which to implement this new lifestyle change. It will help you to track your progress and, in the long term, help you manage and maintain your weight loss and health. A plan allows you to visually see the work you are putting into fasting and to track results. Plus, it will leave you feeling less frazzled when it comes to your fast day and you are unsure of what meals you will be eating and at what times.

Take gradual steps and, eventually, you will be able to master the art of fasting and adapting it to your current lifestyle.

Step One: Create a Monthly Calendar

On a calendar, highlight the days on which you wish to fast, depending on the type of fast you have committed yourself to. Record a start and end time on your fasting days so you know in the days leading up to your fast day what time you plan to begin and finish.

Tick off your days; this will keep you motivated and on track!

Step Two: Record Your Findings

Create a journal for your fasting journey. One or two days before the time, undertake to do your measurements. Weigh yourself first thing in the morning, after you have gone to the restroom, and before breakfast. Also, do not weigh yourself wearing heavy items as they may affect the outcome of the scale.

Measure your height as this figure is related to your BMI (body mass index) result.

Record the measurements around your hips and stomach area, if you wish, you can also measure your upper thighs and arms.

Take a photo of yourself and place it into the journal too; this is not to discourage you but to keep you focused on why you began this journey.

Jot down all of these findings and update them weekly in the journal.

A journal is also the perfect way to express how you are feeling and, of course, what you are most thankful for. A journal is an important way in which to track not just the physical aspects of the diet but also the mental aspects too. Never undertake to doubt yourself; your journal should be a safe space for you to congratulate and to motivate yourself. Leave all the negative thoughts at the door!

Step Three: Plan Your Meals

The easiest way to stick to any eating program is to plan your meals; 500 calorie meals tend to be simple and easy to create but there are also many other more complex recipes for those who wish to spice things up. Who knows, perhaps you stumble across a meal you wish to eat outside of your fasting days.

It is advised that you prepare your meals the day before your fast days; doing this helps you stay committed to the fast and limits food wastage.

Initially, and in the first few weeks, it is suggested that you keep your meal preparation and recipes simple, so as not to overcomplicate the whole process. This also allows you to get used to counting your calories and knowing which foods work to keep you fuller versus those that left you feeling hungrier earlier than later. Be sure to include your meal plan in your journal and on your calendar.

Step Four: Reward Yourself

On the days where you may return to normal eating, it is important to reward yourself. A small reward goes a long way in reminding yourself and your brain that what you are doing has merit and that it should be noticed.

A reward should cater to one of our primal needs; these needs include:

- Self-actualization

- Safety needs

- Social needs

- Esteem needs

- Physiological needs such as food, water, air, clothing, and shelter

Have a block of chocolate, or buy yourself a new item of clothing; do anything that makes your heart happy!

Step Five: Curb Hunger Pains

Initially, you will feel more discomfort when hungry but these feelings will pass. If you do find yourself craving something, sip on black tea or coffee to help you through your day. Coffee is known to alleviate the feelings of being hungry; if you must add sweetener, do so at your discretion. Know that some sweeteners can cause the opposite effect and make you feel hungry.

Step Six: Stay Busy

Keeping busy means that the mind does not have time to dwell on your current state of affairs, especially if you find yourself reaching for a snack bar or cookie.

It is also wise to be implementing some sort of physical activity, even on your fasting days. A 20-minute walk before ending your fasting period will do wonders to help you reach the final stages of the fasting period. It can also uplift your mood when you are feeling frustrated or tense.

Step Seven: Practice Mindful Eating

As mentioned, we are inclined to eat for all sorts of reasons; happy, sad, it does not matter. The problem is that these feelings related to food become habitual, so we aren't really hungry but because we feel good or even off, we seek to tuck into something delicious.

The art of eating mindfully is to not allow these habits to master your life. The concept is simple: teach yourself to look at something, for instance, a piece of cake, and think, "Do I really need it or do I want it for other reasons?" You could decide to have a bite or two and leave the rest, but you may be less inclined to eat the whole slice (or whole cake) if you think mindfully about it.

The art of mindful eating is to revel in the food placed before you. Pay attention to the colors, textures, and tastes. Savor each bite, even when eating an apple.

Your brain gradually begins to rewire itself when it comes to food and when it needs or wants something.

Practice mindful eating by:

- Listen to what your body is telling you; stop eating when you are full.

INTERMITTENT FASTING FOR WOMEN OVER 50

- Only eat when your body signals you to do so; when your stomach growls or if you feel faint or if your energy levels are low.

- Pay attention to what is both healthy and unhealthy for us.

- Consider the environmental impact our food choices make.

- Every time you take a bite of your meal, set your cutlery down.

Step Eight: Practice Portion Control

Controlling portion sizes can be difficult for most; society has also regulated us to what we think is the size of an average portion should be and we have access to supersizing meals too, which does not help those struggling in the weight department. In 1961, Americans consumed 2,880 calories per day; by 2017, they were consuming 3,600 calories, which is a 34% increase and an unhealthy one at that.

To help you navigate how to better portion your food, consider trying the following: when dishing up your food, try the following trick. Half of your plate should consist of healthy fruits and/or vegetables, one quarter should be made up of your starches such as potatoes, rice, or pasta, and the remaining quarter should be made up of lean meats or seafood.

Alternatively, try the following:

- Dish up onto a smaller plate or into a smaller bowl.

- Say no to upsizing a meal if offered.

- Buy the smaller version of the product if available, or divide the servings equally into packets.

- Eat half a meal at the restaurant and take the remaining half to enjoy the following day instead.

- Go to bed early; it will stop any after-dinner eating.

Step Nine: Get Tech Savvy

Modern-day society has plenty to offer us in terms of the apps we can use to help determine the steps we take, the calories we burn, the calories found in our foods, as well as research, information, and motivation for lifestyle changes, especially diets and exercise. The list is endless. There are many apps on the market currently that can help you track your progress with regards to fasting.

The best intermittent fasting apps currently (at the time of writing), and in no particular order are:

- Zero

- FastHabit

- BodyFast

- Fastient

- Vora

- Ate Food Diary

- Life Fasting Tracker

Make use of your mobile device to set reminders for yourself of when to eat, what to eat, and when your fast days are. It works especially well when using it to set reminders for when you should drink water, particularly for those who find it hard to keep their fluids up.

Making the Change

Understand that intermittent fasting is not a diet; it is a lifestyle, an eating plan that you are in control of, and one that is easy to perfect. Before you know it, fasting will become second nature.

When to Start?

Begin today, not tomorrow or after a particular event or gathering. Once you have picked the fast that best suits you, begin with it immediately. Never hold off until a specific day; once you begin, you will gain momentum and it will become something that is part of your day, like many other things that fill up your day. No sweat there!

Measure Your Eating

Three days before you fast, it would be wise to begin to lessen the amount of food you are eating or dishing up less. This helps your body begin to get used to the idea that it doesn't need a whole bowl of food to get what it needs nor to feel full.

Keep up Your Exercise Plan

If you have a pre-existing exercise regime, do not alter it anyway. Simply carry on the way you were before fasting.

Stop, Start, Stop

Fast for hours, and then eat all your calories during a certain number of hours. Consider this as a training period.

Do Your Research

Read up as much as you can about intermittent fasting; this way it will put to rest any uncertainties you might have and introduce you to new ways of getting through a fasting day. Check out recipes that won't make you feel like a rabbit having to chomp on carrots all day if you are stuck with ideas of what to eat.

Have Fun

Lastly, have fun, and see what your body can do, even over 50. It is important to know that just because you are a certain age doesn't mean you are incapable of pursuing a new lifestyle change.

Reward yourself when it is due, track your progress, adjust where it is needed, and get your beauty sleep. This is another secret to achieving overall wellness and happiness.

CHAPTER 12:

Intermittent Fasting & Keto Diet: The Perfect Duo

The ketogenic diet offers many of the same benefits associated with intermittent fasting and fasting, and when done together, most people will experience significant health improvements, including not just weight loss. The ketogenic diet and intermittent fasting allow the body to move from a state where sugar is burned to a state where fat is burned (important flexibility, which in turn promotes optimal cell function and body systems). And although there is evidence that the two strategies work independently, I understand that the combination of the two strategies provides the best results overall.

There are at least two important reasons to favor the pulse approach. Insulin deactivates liver gluconeogenesis, that is, the production of glucose by the liver. When insulin is chronically suppressed for long periods, the liver begins to compensate for its lack by producing more glucose. As a result, your blood sugar starts rising even if you don't eat carbohydrates.

In this case, eating carbohydrates will lower your blood sugar because they activate insulin, which shuts down glucose production in the liver. Long-term chronic deactivation of insulin constitutes an unhealthy metabolic state that can be easily avoided by entering and exiting cyclically from ketosis.

More importantly, in general, many metabolic benefits associated with nutritional ketosis occur during the re-feeding phase. In the fasting phase, the removal of damaged cells and their contents occurs, but the real rejuvenation process takes place during refeeding. In other words, the cells and tissues are rebuilt and their healthy state is restored when the intake of net carbohydrates increases. (Rejuvenation during re-feeding is also one of the reasons why intermittent fasting has so many benefits because you cycle hunger and abundance.)

How to apply cyclic ketosis and fasting

1. Take an intermittent fasting program: eat all meals (from breakfast to lunch, or from lunch to dinner) within an eight-hour time frame each day. Fasting for the remaining 16 hours. Once it becomes a routine, continue implementing the ketogenic diet, and then making it cyclical. You can find comfort in knowing that once you reach the third step you can replenish some of your favorite healthy carbohydrates weekly.

For example, I do it three or four times a year. To simplify this process, gradually reach a point where you fast for twenty hours a day and eat two meals in just four hours. After a month, fasting while consuming only water for five days will not be that difficult.

2. Switch to a ketogenic diet until you generate measurable ketones: the three main stages are: limit the net carbohydrates (total carbohydrates without fiber) from 20 to 50 grams per day; replace the eliminated carbohydrates with healthy fats to obtain 50 to 85% of the daily caloric intake from fats and limit the protein to half a gram for every half kilo of lean body mass. (To determine your lean body mass, subtract your body fat percentage to 100, then multiply that percentage by your current weight.)

Vegetables, which are full of fiber, can be eaten without restrictions. The main sources of carbohydrates that must be eliminated are cereals and all forms of sugar, including fruits rich in fructose. (Healthy net carbohydrates will then be replenished once ketosis is activated.) Examples of sources of healthy fats include avocados, coconut oil, omega 3 derived from oily fish, butter, raw nuts (macadamia nuts and pecans are ideal because they are rich in healthy fats but they contain few proteins), seeds, olives, and olive oil, grass-fed animal products, MCT oil, natural cocoa butter, and pasteurized organic egg yolks.

Avoid all trans fats and polyunsaturated vegetable oils that are not fine. Adding these harmful fats can cause more damage than excess carbohydrates, so just because a food is "high in fat" doesn't mean you should eat it. Keep these portions of net carbohydrates, fats, and proteins until you get into ketosis and your body burns fat as an energy source. To determine that you are ketotic, you can use the ketone test strips, checking that the ketones in your blood are in the range of 0.5 to 3.0 mmol/L.

Remember that precision is important when it comes to portions of these nutrients. In fact, an excess of net carbohydrates will prevent ketosis as the body will first use any available glucose source, being a type of fuel that burns faster. Since it is practically impossible to accurately determine the amount of fat, net carbohydrates, and proteins in all dishes, make sure you have some basic measuring and tracking tools at your fingertips.

3. Once you have verified you are in ketosis, start cycling in and out of ketosis by replenishing high amounts of net carbohydrates once or twice a week: As a general recommendation, the number of net carbohydrates triples during the days you fill up on carbohydrates.

Remember that the body will again be able to effectively burn fat at any time after a couple of weeks or a few months. As already mentioned, entering and exiting cyclically from nutritional ketosis will maximize biological benefits of regeneration and renewal, while at the same time minimizing potential negative sides of continuous ketosis. At this point, even if high or low carbohydrates are given once or twice a week, I would still advise you to be careful about what is healthy and what is not.

Ideally, you should avoid potato chips and donuts, and focus on taking in healthier alternatives such as digestive-resistant starches. The foods rich in net carbohydrates such as potatoes, rice, bread, and pasta all become resistant to digestion when cooked, cooled, and then heated again, and it is a way of making these indulgences a little healthier.

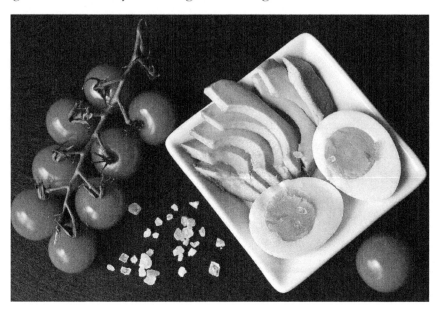

CHAPTER 13:

How Does Intermittent Fasting Help in Weight Loss?

What Is the Mechanism Behind Losing Weight?

If you truly want to understand how you can lose weight or what makes you gain weight, then understanding certain hormonal functions is also important. This, in turn, will also help you understand the working mechanism of intermittent fasting. Now, two very important hormones in your body control the levels of blood glucose, and these are insulin and glucagon. And there is another pair about whom you must have some knowledge and they are brown fat and white fat. You will keep gaining and losing weight and it is quite a natural fluctuation that the human body goes through. To understand this process, having full knowledge of these pairs is essential.

Insulin and Glucagon

You might have already done some research on how insulin is related to your blood glucose or blood sugar levels. But what we are going to discuss here is how any of this is related to gaining weight. Now, the place where insulin is made in your body is none other than the pancreas, and this insulin, in turn, is responsible for maintaining proper levels of blood glucose.

People suffer from hyperglycemia when the levels of glucose in their blood become high. Similarly, they suffer from hypoglycemia when the levels of glucose in their blood become low. When you are eating food, there is a subsequent rise in the levels of glucose in your blood. This is because the food is being digested as a result of which glucose is formed by the transformation of carbohydrates. This glucose is then utilized by the organ systems so that they can get the energy to perform their activities. Now, when you think about carbs, I bet that the first food items that come to your mind are probably something along the lines of pasta and bread, but there are so many veggies and fruits that are rich in carbs as well.

Now, when there is a rise in the levels of glucose in the blood, insulin is released from the pancreas. The task of insulin is to signal the fats, muscles, and liver in your body to start the absorption of glucose from the bloodstream. This is the actual process in which the different organ systems derive energy. When the amount of glucose is more in the blood than what is required, the glucose gets stored in the form of glycogen in the liver. Sometimes, insulin helps in converting excess glucose into fatty acids. The adipose tissues in your body are where the fats are stored.

Now, three things are inhibited by the presence of insulin, and they are as follows: gluconeogenesis, glycogenolysis, and lipolysis. So, lipolysis is when your body engages in the breakdown of fats to derive energy for day-to-day activities. Glycogenolysis is when usable glucose is formed by the breakdown of glycogen. The process is inhibited by the presence of insulin. And lastly, gluconeogenesis is when the non-carbohydrate sources act as the substrate from which glucose is created.

So, we have two hormones working behind the scenes. The three mechanisms mentioned above are set into motion by the presence of glucagon, and these mechanisms are the reason why there is a rise in the levels of glucose in your blood. But the presence of insulin has the capability of inhibiting these mechanisms and then reducing the levels of glucose in the blood.

What Are the Barriers That Women Face When It Comes to Weight Loss?

There was a study that was conducted by the Yale Journal of Biology and Medicine, and in it, it was stated how women are more prone to being obese than men. In fact, the chances of a woman being obese are twice that of a man. Now, if you are wondering, why then here are the reasons :

Hormones

One of the biggest reasons for women being more prone to weight gain is their hormonal makeup. Factors like diet, aging, and stress play a big role in the alteration of hormones like estrogen, cortisol, and progesterone, and obesity is a by-product of all these changes taken together. The reason behind women not being adapted to these hormonal changes is because our diets are being increasingly composed of foods that are highly processed.

Also, the process of storing fat in the body of a woman is influenced by the hormone estrogen, which is also known as the female sex hormone. One of the most common signs of aging in women is that they start gaining weight and losing muscles and the major reason is the reduction in the level of estrogen. An important event in the life of women over the age of 50 is menopause and with menopause comes the reduction of estrogen in the body.

Metabolism

The process of metabolism that is present in women is not the same as that in men, and some differences will show you how it acts as a barrier to weight loss. The amount of lean muscles is more in men than in women and this greater number of lean muscles is one of the reasons why the resting metabolic rate of men is higher. There is a scientific reason behind it too. The efficiency of muscles to burn calories is much more than fats. So, possessing a greater number of lean muscles automatically means that they are going to burn more calories. So, even if a man is

not performing any strenuous physical activity, he will be burning more calories than a woman doing the same thing.

The process becomes worse because the storage of fat is also different between the two genders. The fat, in the case of women, is mostly stored in areas like thighs, buttocks, and hips. And any fitness expert can confirm that these are exactly the regions which need a lot of effort to shed fat from.

Emotions

Yes, no matter how you feel about this one but emotions do play a big role when it comes to weight loss, especially in women. The American Journal of Clinical Nutrition confirms the fact that emotional eating is something that women are more engaging with than men. It was in the year 2013 that this study was published. Some of the findings that this research had are as follows:

• Women are more inclined towards maintaining a diet, but maintaining something consistently for some time also requires an immense amount of motivation and willpower. Both these factors can be adversely affected by fluctuation in emotions that can, in turn, lead to stress. Also, it was found that emotional eating was a case that was more common in those women who were following some kind of diet and not that much common in those who were not following any diet at all. Thus, women need to be more aware of the factors that can cause stress and trigger an emotional eating response.

• Probably the worst part about someone engaging in emotional eating is that they will not go for a healthy smoothie or kale salad in case something is bothering them, or they are utterly depressed. Instead, they will reach out for sugary stuff like ice cream, cookies, and chocolates, all of whom have a lot of calories.

•   Lastly, it is not that much to break out of a pattern of emotional eating. But at the end of the day, emotional eating is nothing but a learned behavior, and such behaviors can be unlearnt with proper effort and willpower. But you have to realize that you are in this vicious cycle and you have to break free otherwise if you go too deep into it, then breaking free will become equally difficult.

Genetics

The genetic makeup of a person is also one of the reasons why they are more prone to obesity than others. For example, if every woman in your lineage tended to be over the average BMI, then there are high chances that you will have the same tendency too. So, no matter how much effort you put into weight loss, these factors will still be working against you.

So, the only thing that you have to do is keep reminding yourself not to expect any results soon. To lower your BMI, one of the key steps to take is to live an incremental lifestyle. But yes, intermittent fasting is an effective tool to help you in your weight loss journey.

Relation Between Weight Loss and Intermittent Fasting

Now that we are talking so much about fat and glucose and the difference between them as a source of energy, you must have understood that even fat is nothing but the body's way of storing energy. To make fat more easily available to your body, there are certain changes taking place in your body during the fasting window. These are all related to the metabolism of the body, and they are explained below:

•   Insulin Levels: The level of insulin in the human body shows an increase whenever you are eating something. In the same manner, the opposite happens when you do not eat food; that is, the level of insulin decreases. And when this happens, the process of fat burning is facilitated.

•   Human Growth Hormone or HGH: The levels of this hormone increase to five or six times their usual amount during the fasting window. The main functions of this hormone include loss of fat and gain in muscles, but apart from this, it helps in a lot of other things as well.

•   Norepinephrine: The fat cells receive norepinephrine when you are on a fast as a message sent by the nervous system. After this, the formation of fatty acids takes place in the body. Then, they serve as an alternative source of fuel to cater to your body's energy requirements.

CHAPTER 14:

Why Is Intermittent Fasting The Best Approach For Weight Loss After 50?

A Step By Step Approach

The best way to approach intermittent fasting is to move step by step. You must never undermine the fact that our lifestyles are heavily centered around food. There are shorter gaps between meals. There is a high amount of carb intake that also aggravates the situation to a great extent.

If you follow a very hard approach from the word GO, you are bound to face adjustment issues. The best approach is to allow the body to adapt to the fasting schedule and let it build the capacity to stay hungry.

Eliminate Snacks

This is something that would come several times in this book. It is a very important thing that you must understand. The root cause of most of our health issues is the habit of frequent snacking.

Snacking leads to 2 major issues:

1. It keeps causing repeated glucose spikes that invoke an insulin response and hence the overall insulin presence in the bloodstream increases aggravating the problem of insulin resistance.

2. It usually involves refined carb and sugar-rich food items that will lead to cravings and you will keep feeling the urge to eat at even shorter intervals.

This is a reason your preparation for intermittent fasting must begin with the elimination of snacks. You can have 2–3 nutrient-dense meals in a day, but you will have to remove the habit of snacking from your routine.

As long as the habit of snacking is there, you'll have a very hard time staying away from food as this habit never allows your ghrelin response clock to get set at fixed intervals. This means that you will keep having urges to eat sweets and carb-rich foods, and you will also have strong hunger pangs at regular intervals.

The solution to this problem is very simple. You can take 2–3 nutrient-dense meals that are rich in fat, protein, and fiber. Such a meal will not only provide you with adequate energy for the day but would also keep your gut engaged for long so that you don't have frequent hunger pangs.

The farther you can stay away from refined carb-rich and sugar-rich food items, the easier you would find it to deal with hunger.

You must start easy. Don't do anything drastic or earth-shattering.

Simply start by lowering the number of snacks you have in a day. The snacks have not only become a need of the body, but they are also a part of the habit. In a day, there are numerous instances when we eat tit-bits that we don't care about. We sip cold drinks, sweetened beverages, chips, cookies, bagels, donuts, burgers, pizzas simply because they are in front of us or accessible. We have made food an excuse to take breaks. This habit will have to be broken if you want to move on the path of good health.

Widen the Gap Between Your Meals

This is the second step in your preparation. You must start widening the gap between your meals. This process needs to be gradual and should only begin when you have eliminated snacks from your routine.

Two nutrient-dense meals in a day or two meals and a smaller meal or lunch comprising of fiber-rich salads should be your goal.

However, you must remember that these two steps must be taken over a long period. You must allow your body to get used to the change. There would be a temptation that it is easy to follow these, and you can jump to the actual intermittent fasting routine, but it is very important to avoid all such temptations as they are only going to lead to failures.

If your body doesn't get used to this routine, very soon, you'll start feeling trapped. You'll start finding ways to cheat the routine. You'll look for excuses to violate the routine, and it very soon becomes a habit. This is the reason you must allow your body to take some time to adjust to the new schedule.

You should remember that intermittent fasting is a way of life. This might slower the results, but it is going to make your overall journey smoother and better.

CHAPTER 15:

Hormonal Health of Women

One of the most dangerous things that women do while they are trying to lose weight is that they ignore the importance of their hormonal health. One of the most significant differences between men and women is the way their bodies treat food. The body of a man doesn't attach too much significance to food. For men, food is just a way to survive. This is in stark contrast to the way the body of a woman treats food. For women, food means much more than simple survival; it is connected to their hormonal balance.

From the time a girl hits puberty to the time she reaches menopause, her body is physically always in a readiness mode to bear a child. Bearing a child is a big responsibility. A child in the womb is a big drain on the energy sources in a woman's body. Once a woman conceives a child, her body tries its best to provide nutrition to the child. This was always not possible through conventional mediums in the past. In the past, women sometimes got food and most of the time didn't.

This can make the survival of the child in the womb difficult. To solve this problem, nature has devised the plan of energy storage inside the body to help the child survive.

This is the reason women have a comparatively higher body fat ratio than men, and they are also more likely to gain fat rapidly. It is not a weakness they have, but a brilliant plan devised by nature for the survival of the coming generations.

Food and Female Hormones Are Connected

The hormones in the body are chemical messengers that help in passing on vital information to the brain. Hormones regulate several crucial functions. If you look closely, the life of a woman is completely dominated by these hormones.

The thyroid and pituitary are two very important glands that secrete most of the hormones. They also regulate the behavior of a woman. These glands are also present in men but don't have that profound impact on them simply because they are not going to bear a child.

Women feel a very strong connection with food and that's why emotional eating, impulsive eating, celebration eating, and all other forms of eating have such strong meanings for women. For women, food is a part of emotional security as it also helps in the regulation and balancing of certain hormones.

Impact of Calorie-Restrictive Diets of Hormonal Balance

Calorie-restrictive diets can harm the hormonal balance in women. It can fill them with a sense of insecurity, void, and unhappiness. Scientific experiments on mice have shown that prolonged calorie restriction can also lead to the shrinking of female reproductive organs, and they may also lose their ability to reproduce effectively.

Strict diets can also cause irregular periods, and they may also face problems in conception. Women on calorie-restrictive diets can also experience strong and sudden mood swings and they may also become more temperamental. Anger, frustration, irritation, hopelessness, temptation, and cravings are some of the strong feelings experienced by women when they are on calorie-restrictive diets.

It is very important to understand that hormonal balance is very important. Without the hormonal balance, the overall health of a woman will always remain compromised. This is the problem most women keep facing all their lives.

In the pursuit of weight loss and a slender body, women compromise on their hormonal health and end up paying in the form of problems like PCOS, thyroid, metabolic disorders, and other reproductive issues.

Intermittent Fasting: A Reliable Way to Lose Weight Without Compromising Hormonal Health

Intermittent fasting is a safe way to lose weight as it doesn't force you to compromise your hormonal health. Intermittent fasting doesn't make you starve for food or limit your calorie intake specifically.

It is a process that allows you to eat reasonably. There are no calorie restrictions.

This eliminates cravings, temptations, and obsessiveness regarding certain food items, and hence your hormones remain in control.

Intermittent fasting is not about what to eat but when to eat. The most important thing in intermittent fasting is to observe abstinence from food for a certain number of hours every day. This period can be easily timed to be your sleep time, and hence severe hunger pangs and cravings can easily be avoided.

CHAPTER 16:

Tips That Will Help Your Weight Loss Process

Drink Water

I've mentioned this before but it bears repeating. Dehydration is something that can derail you off your path pretty quickly. Your body will let go of any excess water it holds in the beginning and you will see a drop in weight. Don't mistake this for fat loss however, it's just water weight.

Despite this water being considered unnecessary, such a sudden release of fluid can trigger dehydration in some people. The thing to do is to play it safe and prevent it from the start. Purchase a water bottle that has markings on it so you know how much water you're drinking throughout the day.

Aim to drink slightly more than your required intake level and monitor yourself for the symptoms of dehydration I listed earlier in the book. Keep in mind that exercise will result in water loss and you should replenish this water as much as possible. You might be tempted to think that energy drinks will do the job but remember that they contain a lot of sugar and aren't the best option for you.

Stick to good ol' water and you'll be fine.

Plan Ahead

Take some time the night before to plan your day ahead. When will your fasting window end and will you be able to eat a meal at that time? When will you cook and do you need to prep? Prepping is something that tends to catch people out for the most part? This is mostly due to it being a habit they haven't practiced before.

Either way, adopt a preventive approach to all the things you need to do and plan everything out. During the day, try to stay active and busy with tasks. This will keep your mind away from food and hunger. The first few times you carry out IF, you will feel hungry.

Remember that this isn't your body feeling hungry. It's simply a reaction to it expecting food then thanks to the way it has been conditioned. In other words, it's clock hunger and isn't real. You can try to drink some water at this time or have a cup of coffee to push it back. Over a week, you'll find that your body will adjust to it and you'll be fine.

Use Coffee and Tea

When clock hunger strikes your best friends will be coffee and tea. Tea is an especially good choice, specifically green tea. Green tea is a great source of antioxidants and helps fights free radicals. Over and above this, drinking fluids helps reduce those hunger pangs that will occur during the first week when you're adopting IF.

Combine IF With Other Protocols

The best thing you can do once you've adjusted to IF is to combine it with a low-carb diet such as the ketogenic diet. This will help you lose fat a lot faster. Keep in mind that the keto diet is not an easy one to follow, especially for vegans. The best approach to take is to ease into it.

You can start by following it on your rest days to see if you're able to make it work. If this is the case, you can expand it to your workout days. Your body will take some time to adjust to the keto diet and to be honest, the diet itself is the subject of an entire book and in the interest of space, I'll restrict myself to a few important points.

The first thing to remember with keto is that your body is going to take some time to adjust from burning carbs to fat. Remember that carbs are the primary source of fuel and your body isn't going to simply flip a switch and start burning fat. There is a transition period and this is often referred to as the keto fog.

During this time, which lasts for a week or so, you will feel less energized and you'll feel as if you're not able to get out of second gear. The fog lasts for a week and once this time passes, your body will be able to burn fat as its primary source of fuel pretty easily. Practicing keto on your non-training days is a good way to get your body used to burn fat as its primary fuel source.

The best way to prepare for keto is to plan ahead of time and make sure your meal prep is on point. Always start with your protein intake and then move to the other macros. It is best to calculate your macros and calories up front and then keep your meals as uniform as possible to help avoid calorie counting becoming overwhelming.

Ease yourself into keto much as you would with IF and you'll find that both protocols combined will make a massive difference to your overall health.

Do Not Binge

A common mistake beginners make is to look at the start of the feeding window as being a free for all as far as food is concerned. At first, this can be hard to resist since you'll look at the fasting period as being a wasteland without any food whatsoever. The reason this point of view develops is that people think of IF as being restrictive.

When I say restrictive, I mean to say that some people think of it as being a protocol where you deny yourself food for a while and need to use your willpower to stop yourself from eating. Here's the thing: Human beings are well designed to fast. Think of how our ancestors lived before we built cities and farms and gave birth to the Kardashians.

Food was scarce and wasn't guaranteed. After all, there isn't any deer in this world that will willingly offer itself up to be eaten. People had to go through periods where there wasn't any food available and they still managed to survive. As I've mentioned previously, we've come to associate the clock with our mealtimes and more often than not we feel clock hunger and not real hunger.

IF is simply bringing you back into your natural eating pattern and is preventing you from going down the rabbit hole of allowing the clock to dictate what your stomach needs.

The other problem is with regards to breakfast. How often has someone wagged their finger at you and said, "Breakfast is the most important meal of the day!" Here's a fun fact for you: That saying was a marketing slogan invented by Kelloggs to sell more cereal. Here's another fun fact: John Harvey Kellogg the founder of the company figured breakfast was the solution to cure the sin of masturbation amongst young people (The Surprising Reason Why Dr. John Harvey Kellogg Invented Corn Flakes, 2020).

No, I'm not making that up! You can see his line of thought. You can't masturbate if you're shoving god-awful cereal into your face, can you? Either way, that's the background story of the so-called "most important meal of the day". There is no proof of any adverse effects of skipping breakfast or of not eating breakfast during the time designated for it (Leangains.com, 2020).

All in all, don't worry about skipping breakfast or even a meal. All that matters are your calories in versus out. Recognize what clock hunger is and get back in touch with your body's needs.

CHAPTER 17:

Foods to Eat & Avoid in Intermittent Fasting

On the off chance that quick weight reduction while expending about boundless measures of fat sounds unrealistic, "reconsider", keto diet fans state. Supporters of the stylish high-fat, low-carb feast plan swear it clears the mind while bringing down the number on the scale. Albeit long haul wellbeing impacts of the eating routine, which requires generally 80% of your everyday calories to originate from fat, are as yet obscure for the normal individual, the Keto diet has for quite some time been utilized to treat youngsters with epilepsy and individuals with diabetes. Yet, the greatest inquiry of everything is how does eating keto diet nourishments cause you to get in shape when you're eating bacon, margarine, and cheddar? Continue perusing for the subtleties, besides, to realize which nourishments you can (and can't!) eat on this eating routine.

Carbs (5%-10% of calories)

Estimated grams of carbs every day dependent on a 2,000-calorie diet: 40

"Definitely constraining your admission of glucose, the typical vitality hotspot for your cells, diminishes insulin emissions in your body. Since low degrees of glucose are coming in, the body utilizes what is put away in the liver and afterward the muscles," says Rania Batayneh, MPH, the creator of The One Diet: The Simple 1:1:1 Formula for Fast and Sustained Weight Loss. After around three or four days, the entirety of the amassed is spent. Nosh on noodles or other high-carb nourishments and you'll send your body once again into glucose-consuming mode; eat nearly nothing and you'll likely feel your vitality hauling. Most keto health food nuts expect to eat between 20 to 50 grams of carbs every day to keep up that ketone-consuming state called "ketosis."

You should expect to score your carbs from high-fiber, water-rich foods grown from the ground to normally help hydration and keep your stomach-related framework murmuring along. Uncertain of whether a produce pick is low in carbs? Reach for alternatives become over the ground (verdant greens, peppers, and stalk-molded vegetables), as opposed to subterranean (root veggies like potatoes, carrots, and parsnips), as they normally offer fewer carbs.

Genuine instances of carb keto diet nourishments:

•Tomatoes

•Eggplant

•Asparagus

•Broccoli

•Cauliflower

•Spinach

•Green Beans

•Cucumber

•Bell peppers

•Kale

•Zucchini

•Celery

•Brussels grows

Protein (10%-20% of calories)

Protein is basic to fabricate muscle cells and consume calories. Eat excessively or excessively little of it as a major aspect of your keto diet nourishment plan and you'll wind up subverting your objectives.

Without carbs and protein, for example, in case you're adhering to the low-carb share of keto and eating more fat and less protein than suggested, your body will go to muscle tissue as fuel. This, thus, will bring down your general bulk and the number of calories you consume very still. Overdose on the protein (following this macronutrient breakdown, that would liken to anything well beyond one six-ounce steak and one four-ounce chicken bosom) you'll put undue strain on your kidneys. Additionally, your body will change over the abundance of protein to starches for fuel. That is the specific inverse objective of the keto diet. Go for around 15% of calories from high-fat protein sources like that underneath. A few, for example, Greek yogurt, eggs, and cheddar give significant nutrients to keep your hair, eyes, and invulnerable framework solid.

While prepared meats like frankfurter and bacon are allowed on the keto diet, I'd prescribe constraining them since they're high in sodium.

Genuine instances of protein keto diet nourishments:

- Chicken, dim meat if conceivable

- Turkey, dim meat if conceivable

- Venison

- Beef

- Salmon

- Sardines

- Tuna

- Shrimp

- Pork

- Lamb

- Eggs

- Natural cheeses

- Unsweetened, entire milk plain Greek yogurt

- Whole milk ricotta cheddar

- Whole milk curds

- Opt for natural, field raised, and grass-took care of, if conceivable, for meat and poultry

Fat (70-80% of calories)

Surmised grams of carbs every day dependent on a 2,000-calorie diet: 165

Here's the place the majority of your admission becomes possibly the most important factor. A few examinations have demonstrated that a higher-fat eating routine can decrease desires and levels of hunger animating hormones ghrelin and insulin. At the point when you're amassing your keto diet nourishment stash, go full-fat. Furthermore, don't worry over the dietary cholesterol content, a factor of how a lot of creature protein you eat, recommends an investigation distributed in The Journal of Nutrition. Rather, center around expending a higher proportion of unsaturated fats (flaxseed, olive oil, nuts) to soaked fats (fat, red meat, palm oil, spread). Since you're devouring a larger part of calories from fat, it's significant to concentrate on filling up with choices that are more averse to stop up your corridors and less inclined to build your disease hazard.

Genuine instances of fat keto diet nourishments:

- Olive oil

- Avocado oil

- Olives

- Avocados

- Flaxseeds

- Chia seeds

- Pumpkin seeds

- Sesame seeds

- Hemp hearts

- Coconuts

- Nuts

- Natural, no-sugar-included nut spreads

What to Avoid

Make it simpler to remain inside the macronutrient system of the keto diet by avoiding these nourishments;

- Beans, peas, lentils, and peanuts

- Grains, for example, rice, pasta, and oats

- Low-fat dairy items

- Added sugars and sugars

- Sugary refreshments, including juice and pop

- Traditional nibble nourishments, for example, potato chips, pretzels, and wafers

- Most natural products, aside from lemons, limes, tomatoes, and little segments of berries

- Starchy vegetables, including corn, potatoes, and peas

- Trans fats, for example, margarine or other hydrogenated fats

- Most alcohols, including wine, brew, and improved mixed drinks

CHAPTER 18:

How The Woman's Body Changes?

The body does not stop changing throughout our lives. Age and genetics are primarily responsible for these changes, although not the only ones. External factors such as tobacco, alcohol, poor diet, or excessive sunbathing are determinants for the deterioration of our health over the decades.

In the case of women, the number of hormones that we have determines the evolution of our bodies over the decades. Fertility is also key to understanding the changes that occur. "Between the decades of the 20s and 60s, the woman undergoes a series of important changes, both hormonally and physically, as a result of menstrual cycles, pregnancies, and other derivatives of reproductive aging".

At 20 years old

During this decade, the woman is full of energy and performance and we enjoy a baseline health status. The body adapts to our rhythm of life and we perform better physically.

Genetics is a fundamental factor that determines endogenous aging however, everything takes its toll. As much as at 20 years the skin is full of collagen, a weekend of excesses on the beach or smoking daily are points that accumulate against the epidermis and time. "If a person with a genetic predisposition to have a thinner dermis or lighter skin, also smokes, sunbathes and excessive gesticulation may have wrinkles in the 20s."

Creating good eating and exercise habits while avoiding alcohol and smoking, as well as paying attention to eating disorders and attending gynecological exams annually.

As for the skin, during this decade and the third, the woman loses the brightness of adolescence and therefore must start using moisturizers, which should subsequently be rich in alpha-hydroxy acids.

During the second decade, the woman is in the fullness of her sexual development by ovarian activity. The secretion of hormones such as estrogen and progesterone play a fundamental role in the menstrual cycle and fertility.

At birth, our ovaries have a million oocytes and will no longer be produced. In each menstrual cycle, they are discarded, so as time progresses the possibility of becoming a mother decreases until menopause arrives. Between the ages of 15 and 25, the probability of becoming pregnant in each cycle is 40 %. During this time, contraceptive treatments should be taken into account to avoid unwanted pregnancy as well as assistance in the transmission of infectious diseases.

At 30 years old

From the age of 30, there is a decrease in metabolism, which means that, if we do not exercise, we burn fewer calories per minute naturally.

The specialist Concepción de Lucas points out that if you also lead a sedentary lifestyle, with work stress or poor diet, your physical condition can get worse.

Also, this is the decade in which most Spanish women have their first child: the average is 32 years old. The expert points out that this moment is key for women. "In this decade, muscle tone is lost and, with pregnancy, the body can undergo significant changes, with increases and decreases in weight, body volume, and muscle sagging."

It is also common to observe adult acne, which usually appears in the jaw area and that is due to excessive sensitivity of the skin of that area to hormonal changes and that can be treated with oral contraceptive treatments or oral recurrences (not indicated for pregnant women since it can cause alteration is in the fetus) or synthetic, as dermatologist María Teresa Truchuelo explains. This type of acne may also be due to disorders such as the polycystic ovary or the use of overly fatty cosmetics.

From the age of 30, expression wrinkles begin to appear in the areas where we are most gesturing, such as between the eyebrows or the eye area, with bags and crow's feet.

The specialist recommends using moisturizers and containing active ingredients such as the aforementioned alpha hydroxy acids, which seek to reshape the skin, vitamin C, and niacinamide.

You have to maintain good eating and exercise habits, go to gynecological exams annually and do health checks to monitor cholesterol, weight, visual and auditory acuity, and the early detection of diseases and pathologies.

From the age of 35, the woman's fertility decreases and it is increasingly difficult to get pregnant, so gynecologists advise not to delay motherhood beyond this age because, in addition to having to resort to assisted reproduction techniques, They add the risks of having abortions, hypertension, diabetes, and deformations or alterations in the fetus. From the age of 40, the probability of pregnancy in each cycle is 25 %.

At 40 years old

During the fourth decade of our life, a series of changes in our physiognomy begin to occur. The fat that predominated in the buttocks and legs for possible breastfeeding begins to redistribute in the abdomen, increasing the risk of cardiovascular disease.

Also, decrease muscle mass and tone and increases sagging in arms and legs, especially if we do not exercise.

The level of hormones drops and the woman is moving away from her period of greatest fertility.

The skin loses elasticity and sunspots begin to develop like antigens, which are more marked on the lighter skins. "Expression wrinkles intensify, and facial volumes begin to vary. The expert recommends anti-spot lasers, botulinum toxin for expression wrinkles, and hyaluronic acid to treat wrinkles of the nasogenial groove and volume loss.

Good eating habits and exercise will contribute to a better menopausal transition in the future, as Lucas warns. The specialist indicates that, from the age of 40, the tendency to suffer from hypertension and cholesterol, pathologies that are also observed in men, rises.

Besides, the intervertebral discs are compressed, and it is normal for spine pain, loss of muscle tone to increase, and osteoporosis or loss of bone mass. "It is important that young women prevent their appearance by performing a diet rich in calcium and muscle strength exercises." This serves to condition the muscles, make them stronger and stronger. It also strengthens the union of muscle with a bone through tendons.

From 45-50 years old, women can begin to notice hot flashes, irritability, difficulty sleeping, vaginal dryness, decreased libido, and alterations in menstruation; "We are in premenopause, " explains Esparza, who advises seeing it as" a natural stage in women, "which must be normalized and treated if necessary, to reduce symptoms. "We must not fear it, or there are methods to prevent it, simply accept it as another stage as a person and as a woman."

From the age of 45, early menopause can also occur, which usually occurs between 50 and 55 years.

From 50 years old

During the 50s, women begin to suffer from menopause, which is the absence of menstruation for more than 12 months and is due to the permanent cessation of follicular function. Its diagnosis is clinical and retrospective when 12 months have elapsed since the last period without any menstrual bleeding.

Lucas's conception clarifies that "there are no clear guidelines on how to deal with it because each woman has different experiences, but most of the changes in their bodies are related to it."

During this period, the alteration in the distribution of body fat continues, the appearance of the skin in terms of elasticity and hydration worsens, vaginal dryness and other mucous membranes that can cause pain during sexual intercourse are experienced, muscle tone decreases and muscle damage deteriorates. bones of the spine, joints, or osteoarthritis problems appear.

"It also increases cardiovascular risk, sleep and memory disorders influenced by the gradual loss of estrogen," explains the specialist, adding that lifestyle changes can cause several mood changes: " during this stage, it is normal to suffer more anxiety, depression and a decrease in mood. "

The woman who is in the fifth decade may also notice that she loses pubic and axillary hair, undergoes changes in hair and skin, or increases in body weight.

Menopause causes that, between 50 and 60 years, the woman's skin experiences many alterations. "The decrease in estrogen that occurs at this time in the woman's life leads to a thinning of the skin and dehydration, which causes wrinkles to intensify and 'sagging' of structures."

Acclimatizing the body to the symptoms of menopause by reducing body temperature with light clothing and drinking cold drinks, as well as exercising regularly to prevent osteoporosis. Proper nutrition, doing controlled breathing exercises, and going to gynecological exams and other medical check-ups are also tips to keep in mind during this stage and during the sixth decade of our life.

The specialist also recalls that "throughout the woman's life, the gynecologist must be present, adapting her actions to the different health and reproductive status."

At every stage of the woman, physical changes, as well as psychological changes, occur, and that the specialist must be a foothold to ask constantly. "These are vital phases that must be accepted and lived. Every change you don't understand or doubt you have; you will have your gynecologist to solve them."

CHAPTER 19:

Can Intermittent Fasting Extend a Woman's Fertility?

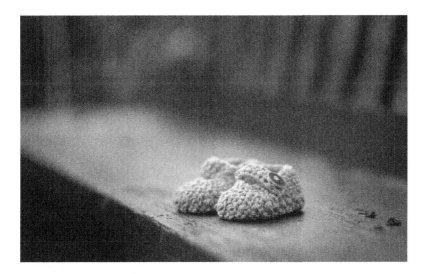

For women over 50, this may not be a huge issue. However, it is still important to keep in mind how intermittent fasting can affect women's bodies, especially if you wish to recommend this diet to a younger woman. If intermittent fasting can extend female fertility is a topic that has been asked for a while, but recent studies that were carried out have now shed light on this question. It is no secret that aging causes the reduction of the quality and quantity of eggs.

There have been a few recent studies that were carried out in mice, whereby their calorie intake was reduced by 40%. This significantly improved their egg quality and showed that just a few of their eggs contained abnormal chromosomes when they got to their reproductive years. This is not the same as their counterparts that were allowed to eat as much as they wanted. It is the abnormalities in eggs that usually cause congenital disabilities and raise the risk of having miscarriages. The study further showed that mice that underwent intermittent fasting could produce more eggs than the mice that ate as they liked. Restriction of calories also increased the survival of the offspring after birth and also prolonged their reproductive life span. This study concluded that when you manipulate nutrition, you can adjust the signal pathways.

Another study that was carried out on worms showed that during intermittent fasting, the worms put reproduction on hold. It helped them to terminate the sex cells that existed to be able to generate healthy eggs. The lifespan of the worms that underwent intermittent fasting was greatly extended. Human beings may go through the same process, but tests are yet to be done. The PPAR gamma is the protein that scientists say might do the job of controlling the rate at which ovulation occurs. The studies are also not clear about the amount of calorie restriction needed to turn on such systems in human beings. Many fertility problems could be solved if only the identification and manipulation of signaling molecules could be made. This could even extend the reproductive life span of a woman.

Fasting has been said to improve the chances of couples that have been trying to conceive through in vitro fertilization but were never successful. Fertility specialists found out that intermittent fasting can alkalize the blood system, remove synthetic hormones, and cleanse the liver. They also said that when you fast, the body's natural hormone process is rebooted. The calorie intake of people who take the time or find it hard to conceive is usually evaluated. If it is high, with the help of a nutritionist, they are started on intermittent fasting. This will not only get rid of toxins in the patient's body, but it will also help them to get closer to their required body mass index. Intermittent fasting will cause the rebalancing of hormones, and the liver will metabolize any excess hormones. Fasting will also cause the regeneration of all organs in the body, and issues like inflammation are reduced. It will also boost the immune system and cause the nervous system to rest hence making the reproductive system ready for conception.

In males, intermittent fasting can greatly increase the sperm count of men who suffer from fertility issues. It can also boost the levels of testosterone hormones in those who do not suffer from fertility issues.

CHAPTER 20:

How To Overcome Down Moments?

When it comes to one's ultimate health and desire to achieve the targets, controlling appetite, and keeping healthy food is important. Intermittent fasting will help you accomplish this, but although certain individuals can fast with very little problem for long stretches, some people can find it a bit more challenging, particularly when they first start.

There is a set of ideas to help you out that one can use to get the best results and make the ride a little smoother.

Start the Fast After Dinner

One of the best advice one can offer is when you do regular, or weekly fasting is to begin the fast after dinner. Using this ensures you're going to be sleeping for a good portion of the fasting time. Especially when using a daily fasting method like 16/8

Eat More Satisfying Meals

The type of food one consumes affects their willingness to both the urge to complete the fast and what you crave to eat after the fast.

Too much salty and sugary foods with making you hungrier rather than consume meals that are homey satisfying and will help you lose weight

• Morning eggs or oats porridge

• A healthy lunch of chicken breast, baked sweet potato, and veggies.

- After the workout, drink a protein milkshake.

- Then you end the day in the evening with an equally impressive dinner.

Control Your Appetite

Without question, while fasting, hunger pangs can set in from start to end. The trick as this occurs is to curb your appetite, and with Zero-calorie beverages that help provide satiety and hold hunger at bay before it's time to break the fast, the perfect way to do this is. Examples of food to consume are

- Sparkling water

- Water

- Black tea

- Black coffee

- Green tea

- Herbal teas and other zero-calorie unsweetened drinks

Stay Busy

Boredom is the main threat. It is the invisible assassin who, bit by bit, creeps in to ruin the progress, breaking you down steadily and dragging you downwards.

For a second, think about it. How often boredom has caused you to consume more than you can, intend to, or even know that you are. Hence try to plan your day.

Stick to A Routine

Start and break your fast each day at regular times. Consuming a diet weekly where you finish similar items per day. Meal prepping in advance. Making a plan allows things easier to adhere to the IF schedule, so you eliminate the uncertainty and second-guessing the process until you learn what works for you and commit to it every day. Follow-through is what one has to do.

Give Yourself Time to Adjust

When one first starts intermittent fasting, odds are you're going to mess up a couple of times; this is both OK and natural. It's just normal to have hunger pangs. This doesn't mean that you have to give up or that it's not going to be effective for you. Alternatively, it's a chance to learn, to ask whether or how you messed up, and take action to deter it from occurring again.

Enjoy Yourself

Let yourself enjoy the process. No one starts at the pro level, so you should go out with your friends and attend those birthday parties as well.

CHAPTER 21:

Common Mistakes

Intermittent Fasting is a great process that can bring exemplary health effects. However, any process can only work efficiently if its execution is right, and silly mistakes are not made in it.

Pay Attention to Macronutrients

This is one of the most important things to remember. The people who are suffering from obesity simply want to get rid of this malice. They are ready to barter anything for it. They dream of a slender figure as the ultimate goal, and this is where they become susceptible to make some of the most fatal mistakes.

Intermittent fasting or any form of dieting or calorie-restrictive routine would put certain restrictions on you. Intermittent fasting doesn't put a cap on the amount of food you can eat or its type. However, that doesn't mean you can eat a lot. In most cases, you will have only 7–8 hours in reality to eat anything that you want. Although it may look like a lot of time, you would find that the time for the final meal of the day approaches much before the previous meal has got digested. Missing that meal may mean that you'll have to go without food till the next meal. Therefore, the amount of food you can eat gets limited.

Other calorie-restrictive routines put an explicit cap on the amount and type of food you can have. These things have a profound impact on your health. You may experience weight loss, but that doesn't mean that you are getting healthy.

Your body can only get healthy when it is getting all the macro and micronutrients in the right quantity. It also needs vitamins and minerals. Getting all that while consuming limited calories can be difficult. If you don't pay proper attention here, you will end up with nutrient deficiencies.

You may get a slender frame, but you will be battling with more problems than you started with.

The best way to counter this problem is to have a properly balanced diet. Intermittent fasting allows you a proper chance to do so as it doesn't put restrictions on the quantity and types of food items you can have.

The best way to pass this trick with qualifying marks is to have a very balanced meal. Your meals should be high in fat, moderate in protein, and low in carbs.

Before you begin to question the credibility of the suggestion, I would like to clarify some misconceptions:

Fat Is Not Bad

There is a popular misconception that eating fat is bad. Fat is the building block of life. Fat, in general, is not bad. Trans fat or the poor-quality fat that we get in processed food is bad. Fat in itself is a form of compact energy. Our body doesn't classify food as fat, protein, or cholesterol. Everything that you eat gets processed and is broken down as calories. This means that fat would get converted to glucose as well, and so would happen with carbs. The benefit of eating fat is that you will be able to get more calories in a single meal in comparison to carbs.

Fat is very compact in nature and has almost double the number of calories per gram when compared to carbs. So if you get 8 calories per gram of carbs, you'll get 16 from fat. Protein is heavier and has more calories than carbs. This means that if you consume a high-fat-low carb diet, you can get more calories and that even if you have fewer meals in a day, you will not get energy deficient.

Fat should be consumed in greater quantities. You should select high-quality fat. The same goes for protein. You can get protein from animals and cereals, and it would help you in muscle building and staying fit. The biggest advantage of having a high-fat, moderate protein, low-carb diet is that it doesn't make you feel hungry very often. Fat and protein content in your meals would help you in transitioning from one meal to the other easily without facing the need to have snacks.

Fat and protein-rich diets also contain a lot of minerals and vitamins. However, the highest part of minerals and vitamins, and fiber should be obtained from carbs. You should consume a lot of leafy green vegetables, salads, whole grain foods. Leafy greens are bulky and but they do not weigh much. They don't add too many calories to your system, but they provide most of the vitamins, minerals, phytonutrients, antioxidants, and trace minerals required by your body. You can have leafy green vegetables as much as you want without worrying about calories.

This is a part that you should never undermine in your pursuit to have a slender figure. If you ignore your health, the weight would come back faster than you can lose it.

You must always remember that you need to be healthy to fight weight, and it isn't the other way around. The people who lose their weight drastically without a solid base are called sick and not healthy.

You must never forget the macronutrients in your meal as they would become the pillars of your health.

Don't Get Greedy in the Feasting Windows

Food has its own temptation. It looks like the most alluring thing in the world when you have been deprived of it for a long time. This would happen to you too. But you mustn't get greedy at such times and lose control. You must properly get off your fasting windows.

The biggest mistake people make is they eat a lot after breaking their fast. This can cause several problems, and poor digestion is one among them. In the fasting state, the gut gets to stay away from food for extended periods, and hence it can get a bit dry. Stuffing it with heavy food can cause problems. The best way to begin the day is to start with liquid food and then transition to semi-solid and solids.

You should, besides, mind the quantity of food that you eat. Our brain takes much longer to understand the leptin signals that you are full. By the time your brain tells you that you are full, you would have already overeaten. The best way out is to either eat slowly as this would give your brain the time to assess your satiety levels. You can also stop eating when you feel that you are 80% full. Generally, by this time, you would have eaten your fill. If you want to test this, you can wait for a while after feeling 80% full, and you'd find that you are no longer feeling hungry. It happens as the fat cells can properly communicate to the brain that it doesn't need to eat anymore.

Don't Try to Rush the Process

Slow and steady wins the race. This is an adage we all have heard, but most of us fail to believe it. We want quick results, and for that, we are ready to make the jumps. However, this is not how the body works. Your body makes the transition very slowly. It needs the time to adjust to any kind of change, positive or negative, and the same would happen even in the case of intermittent fasting.

If you want to succeed with the process, you must ensure that you stick to every stage for some time. You must give your body the required time to adjust. There would be decades-old habits that would need to change, and it can be difficult for your body at times.

Fasting in men and women is completely different. Men have a very rugged system, and it doesn't get affected by a bit extended fasting schedule. However, it isn't the case with women. If you try to jerk your system a bit harder, it can affect your health adversely. Your hormonal system may go for a spin, and it may take very long for it to normalize. A woman's body reacts very differently to stress signals, and hence caution and patience are essential.

Start with the easiest process and give your body the time to adjust to the small breaks. Once it gets used to a certain amount of break, try to extend it a bit slowly. Don't do anything very fast. Always go step by step, and you will get your goal easily and without unnecessary difficulties.

Perseverance is the Key

Impatience is a big problem in people battling with weight. There is no fault of theirs as they are already under great pressure. Most people trying to lose weight have already faced disappointment with other weight loss measures, and hence they want to see the results fast to believe them. They are not ready to wait very long to get the results.

This is a point where problems can occur. Intermittent fasting is not any wonder-process. It is a wonderful process, but it doesn't work by magic. It tries to correct the problems that may have reached their current state of development in decades, at least.

It would take some time for the results to come. You will have to work patiently and not lose hope while the results come. If you quit in between, you wouldn't be able to know if you were making any progress or not. It isn't a process that works overnight. It would require you to take the leap of faith and invest your time and energy into it.

Don't Frame Unrealistic Expectations

We all like to dream big, and that is a good thing. However, we must also remain grounded in reality. This will help in accepting the facts and save a lot of disappointments. Many times we are so engrossed with the imaginary expectations that we fail to recognize the gifts we get. If weight loss is your goal, then think of the amount of time you are ready to devote, the lengths to which you can go for it, and the medical conditions you are facing. Without considering all these facts, expecting a complete makeover would be absurd. If you have made such expectations, then you will not even be able to enjoy the weight loss you are observing. Your expectations would overshadow the results. You must remain realistic.

CHAPTER 22:

New Healthy Habits

Before you begin fasting, there are some things that you will want to do to prepare yourself. It may be difficult mentally and physically, especially if you are new to fasting. Your mindset will become very important as you are fasting, especially the longer you fast at one time. Getting yourself into the proper mindset before you begin will help you to stay focused while you are fasting.

Ensure you Are Fasting in a Healthy Way

When it comes to fasting, it is important to ensure that you approach it in a way that will be beneficial for our health, and that will not do more harm than good.

Firstly, you want to maintain flexibility with yourself and your body when fasting. If you are not feeling well as you are trying to fast, don't be afraid to eat a small amount on your fast days. This is especially true at the beginning when you first introduce fasting into your diet. If you try a water fast for example, and you feel lightheaded and weak, you may decide that you want to instead try an intermittent fasting method like 5/2 which would allow you to eat on your fast days, but in a greatly restricted amount. If you have your mindset on 24-hour water fast, then try the 5/2 method a few times before you try the full water fast to get your body comfortable with reduced amounts of food first.

Increase your Water Intake

As I mentioned, dehydration can accompany fasting since much of our water intake throughout the day comes from the food we eat, like fruits or vegetables. If you are feeling like you are dehydrated while fasting (dry mouth, headache), it is important to increase your water intake. You will also want to ensure you drink enough water each time you fast afterward. The recommendation is about two liters per day, but of course, this depends on your body size. In general, eight glasses of water that are about eight ounces each should give you enough water to be hydrated but when fasting, this must increase to about nine to thirteen glasses. This works out to be between two and three liters of water.

Pay Attention to your Body

If you are feeling very unwell while you are fasting, it is important to know when to stop fasting. It is normal to feel fatigued, hungry, and maybe irritable when you fast, but you may want to stop your fast if you feel completely unwell. To be safe, for your first few times fasting, keep the duration shorter, and work your way up to the desired amount of time. Also, keep some food on you in case you need to eat something due to low blood sugar or feeling unwell. Remember that you are fasting to take care of your body and your health and it should not make you feel worse.

Increase Protein Intake

Ensuring that you eat enough protein while fasting will have numerous benefits for you. Protein takes longer to digest, which means that the energy you get from protein will be longer lasting than the energy you get from other sources like carbohydrates- which are used up quite quickly. Eating enough protein will help to keep your hunger at bay, especially if you are doing the 5/2 method or a method where you will eat small amounts on your fasting days. This will keep you from having an energy "crash" similar to a sugar crash after you have quickly used up the sugars you have ingested.

Select the Foods you Eat Wisely

When you do break your fast or when you are eating small amounts on fasting days, choose the foods you eat wisely. You want to properly prepare your body to fast and keep it healthy while you do so. In addition to eating enough protein, you want to make sure that the other foods you eat are real, whole foods. Whole foods are those which are as close to those found in nature as possible. These are things like meats, vegetables, fruits, fish, eggs, and legumes. This will give you all of the nutrients you need to stay healthy. Eating fast food and processed foods on the days that you are not fasting will leave you feeling tired and without energy, especially if you are fasting the next day or have fasted the day before.

Consider Supplementation

Supplementing may be very beneficial and even necessary when fasting to maintain and improve health. Some essential nutrients and minerals that your body would greatly benefit from like Omega-3's or iron may be difficult to get in adequate amounts if you are fasting. For this reason, supplementing them may benefit you in terms of keeping you feeling healthy and energetic, as well as keeping your brain functioning to its full potential. You can take specific nutrients on their own in pill form or you can opt for a multivitamin that will include all of the most essential vitamins and minerals for overall good health.

Avoid Over-Doing it in the Beginning

Keeping your exercise levels to a minimum while fasting is often necessary as your body will not have as many readily available sugars or carbohydrates to provide you with the quick energy needed for a workout. This is especially important if you are beginning a fasting regimen for the first time.

Your body will need time to adjust to fasting without being extra drained from working out as well. If you are planning to increase your levels of autophagy through a combination of fasting and exercise, wait until your body has adapted to your fasting routine before adding in the exercise portion of the plan.

When Not to Fast

There are times when fasting is not recommended for a person, no matter how used to fasting they may be. If your fasting day comes around and you are feeling any of the following symptoms, fasting that day will not be advisable for you. Knowing when to decide not to fast is important for your health and wellbeing.

If you are feeling sick, including nausea, diarrhea, and general feelings of sickness, take that day or the next few days off of fasting until you are feeling one hundred percent better. Your body needs all of the nutrition it can get while it is trying to fight off sickness and fasting will be taxing to the body, which will make it very difficult for it to fight off the illness.

Things to Take Note of to Ensure Success

Before you begin to fast, as with anything else you set out to do in life, it is important to be aware of your objectives and your motivations for doing it in the first place. It is unlikely that you are doing anything in life without a reason or a motivation for doing so, and if you think you are then maybe your objective is there in the back of your mind somewhere. Think about your objective before you begin, because when you are in the middle of your fast, you will need to look to that objective or motivation to keep you from changing your mind right then and there and breaking your fast for a doughnut.

The Biggest Obstacle: Your Mind

Everybody's objective will differ slightly and will likely be quite personal to them. Maybe you want to reduce your risk of cancer because it runs in your family. Maybe you have been obese for the majority of your life, and you are trying this as a means of weight loss and health improvement. Maybe you heard about it and challenged yourself to try it for a few months to see how it feels. Whatever your objective, writing it down will help to solidify it and make it real. Then, when you are wondering why on earth you decided to put yourself through this on the first day of your fast, you can look at that objective that you wrote down and it will re-inspire you to continue. When it comes to mindset, being aware of your motivation is extremely beneficial.

Your Expectations

By expecting that there will be some uncomfortable side-effects like hunger and irritability, you can greet them with the feeling of "Oh hello, I have been expecting you." Rather than "Oh no I am feeling so terrible what is going on?" If you are not surprised that you will feel a little bit uncomfortable while your body adapts to your fast, you will be able to greet it rather than fighting it, which will make you much more comfortable with it all.

It is important to recognize when fasting that this is a choice you are making for your health, your body, or whatever specific objective you have. You must recognize that this is a choice you are consciously making and that you have decided to go through these times of fasting to later receive the benefits. If you lose sight of the fact that this is a choice you are making, you may begin to feel like a victim or like the universe is punishing you. This victim mindset will only make things harder for you. By taking responsibility for your decision too fast, you will not allow yourself to slip into this negative mindset and will instead feel confident and in control of your decision. This will help you to view things through the lens of appreciation rather than deprivation like I outlined above.

Your Emotions while Fasting

You can prepare as much as you like, but while you are fasting, you could meet some unexpected feelings. Challenging your body and mind often brings up many feelings for us, as it puts us in a state of self-reflection and deep thought. This is normal. Think about if you decided to run a marathon. While running, as your legs desperately want to give up and your body is tired, your mind will likely go to some deep places that they do not go when you are going about your regular daily duties. Fasting is similar to the marathon in this way as it can be very challenging for both the body and the mind.

When emotions come up during your fast, it is important to know what to do with them. The first step is to acknowledge them. By acknowledging these emotions, you can tap into them and examine them in more depth. The next step is to write them down. This can be a very quick note of how you are feeling or what the most challenging part is for you. By writing it down, you are processing this emotion and you can address it instead of pushing it away. When we push our emotions away, they do not go away; they just go dormant for a short period only to come up later. By addressing them, you can examine what is going on inside of you.

CHAPTER 23:

The Right Mindset When Starting IF

When setting out on your intermittent fasting journey, it's important to keep in mind that success is built on several good practices.

The best part is that these secrets are really easy to implement into your routine. So, don't be afraid to give them a try.

The Difference between Needing and Wanting to Eat

It is of the utmost importance for you to recognize when you are really hungry and when you think you are hungry.

There Is a Huge Difference Here

Often, we fall into the trap of eating without actually being hungry. If you are guilty of this, it's time that you started noticing what triggers these cravings. For instance, if you overeat when you are anxious, then it might be a good idea for you to pay close attention to these instances. That can make a significant difference in your overall success.

Eat Only When Needed

When you can recognize when you eat without being hungry, you begin to create a discipline in which you eat only when needed. The easiest way to do this is to build a schedule and then stick to it. Building a rather strict schedule will help you accustom your body to eating only when really needed. This approach will go a long way in helping you stretch your fasting periods.

Hydration Is Essential

Throughout this book, we've talked about how essential it is to hydrate during fast days. You need to make sure that you drink plenty of water. While plain water is perfectly healthy, it should also be mentioned that fruit and vegetable juices are a great source of nutrition.

Ideally, you would consume these juices without any added sugar. Generally speaking, most fruits and vegetables have very few calories. So, you won't blow your calorie budget during fast days. Moreover, most fruits don't have a high glucose content. For instance, apples and lemons don't have much glucose. However, oranges and bananas do. Thus, you want to stick to apple juice and lemon water while cutting down a bit on orange juice. If you can get fresh oranges and squeeze them, you could build a winning formula without consuming needless sugar.

Take Things Slowly

To make this easier, you could use the following rule of thumb. If you are planning to fast on a Monday, you could ramp down your meals, starting with Sunday's lunch. For example, a wholesome lunch (not overdoing it) followed by a very light dinner roughly two hours before bedtime will help you set yourself up for success. Then, consume plenty of water upon getting up on Monday morning. This will keep you full throughout the early morning. Next, make a plan to consume some fruit or non-fat, unsweetened yogurt. This should give you the caloric intake you need. Assuming you are doing a 12–hour fast, plan to have a very light lunch. That way, you won't be burdening your digestive system following the fast. Lastly, you can have a normal dinner, but without overdoing it. The next day, you can go about your usual eating habits.

With this approach, you will never go wrong. You will always feel comfortable at all times during your fasting days.

Cut down on Carbs and Sugar Even on Non-fast Days

During non-fast days, you are free to have your usual eating regimen. However, it's best to cut down on sugar and carbs since being hooked on these will make it very difficult for you to get through a fasting period. Folks who try to fast while seriously hooked on sugar and carbs often feel anxious and edgy. They even suffer from mild to serious withdrawal symptoms.

So, the best way to go about it is to cut down on your sugar intake well before attempting to go on a full fast. For instance, you can cut down on your portion sizes roughly two weeks before attempting to do your first fast. That way, you can begin the detoxing process while avoiding any nasty withdrawal symptoms.

Keep Track of Your Achievements

We're going old school here. Keep track of your achievements by using a regular notebook. There is something about writing things down on paper that makes it highly personal. When you do this, you can see how you have been progressing. Make sure to write down the date and the length of each fast. Also, include some notes about the things that went right and the things that didn't go right. That way, you can see how your intermittent fasting regimen has been affecting you both positively and negatively.

Over time, you can look back to see the progress you've made. That's why journaling can be one of the most important things you can do to give yourself the boost you need, especially when you're feeling depressed. We don't recommend using note-taking or journaling apps on your phone or tablet, as they tend to be quite impersonal. Also, a notebook or journal is a very personal item. Please note that this is a very personal journey. As a result, chronicling your accomplishments will allow you to keep things closer to your heart.

CHAPTER 24:

Dealing with Unpleasant Side Effects

H ere is how to deal with some of the common negative side effects you will likely encounter as you start your new eating habits.

Hunger

One of the first not-so-fun and most obvious results of fasting is hunger. This side effect is difficult because going without food longer than your body is conditioned to will result in an uncomfortable desire for anything to eat. All your life, you have programmed your body to expect food at certain times throughout the day. It would be weird if you suddenly change your eating pattern, and your body accepts the change without putting up at least a little resistance. If your body doesn't get food at the time it normally does, a hormone called ghrelin—the hunger hormone—will start acting up to remind you that you should supply your body with food. This "acting up" or reminder to eat at your usual time will continue until your brain convinces ghrelin to accept your new eating schedule. But until then, you will likely feel intense hunger but don't worry it will pass. You will need to tap into your reserve of mental strength to stay committed to your course.

To effectively handle hunger pangs, drink more water, or any qualifying beverage on intermittent fasting. Doing so will help to suppress hunger pangs. Quite often, the feeling of hunger is not necessarily an indication that you are hungry; it might be a slight dip in your blood sugar level–something that water or other non-calorie liquids can take care of.

To help delay hunger on your fasting days or during the fasting window (depending on the type of fasting regimen you choose to follow), ensure that you include adequate amounts of healthy fats, carbs, and proteins in your meals before commencing your fast. Also, during your fast, try to keep your mind off food. Combining low-impact exercises with fasting can help give you the boost you need to go through your day without feeling too uncomfortable. Getting enough sleep will also help you throughout the day; there is nothing that will upset your day more than lack of sleep at night and having to fast. That is an open invitation for fatigue and hunger!

Frequent Urination

As with hunger, it is also expected to experience an increase in the number of times you urinate. There is no mystery here as intermittent fasting requires that you increase your intake of water and other liquids to stay hydrated. This will in turn increase the frequency of urination. Keep drinking your water and don't avoid bathroom visits. Holding it for too long can weaken your bladder muscles and trying not to drink water will soon make you dehydrated and provide the next side effect– both bad!

Headaches

Intermittent fasting can make your blood sugar take a nosedive. This introduces stress on your body, your brain will release stress hormones, and you will likely experience some degree of headache. Dehydration can lead to headaches during intermittent fasting as your body is telling you it lacks adequate water.

To reduce the occurrence of headaches, try to minimize stress on your body. It is okay to exercise during fasting, but excessive exercise can trigger a large amount of stress. Also, try to keep your body hydrated at all times by drinking enough water. But don't chug water in a rush and don't drink water excessively. Too much water can result in an imbalance in your mineral and body water ratio.

Cravings

It is normal to experience more than usual cravings for food during your fasting window. This is a biological and psychological response to the feeling of deprivation that is often associated with going without food. And because your body is all out to get glucose, you might notice that you crave more sugar or carbohydrates. These cravings don't mean that you are less committed to your goals. Rather, cravings happen to remind you that you are human. Even ardent practitioners of intermittent fasting experience cravings from time to time.

When you start craving for something, remind yourself of your goal and distract yourself from food-related topics. Keep your mind engrossed with other non-food-related activities such as hobbies, talking a walk in nature, or going to sleep for a while. During your eating window, you can treat yourself to a healthy bite of what you crave to minimize the intensity of the craving or longing. Remind yourself during your fasting window that you will soon eat what you long for, so there's no need to dwell on it or giving it too much thought when it is not yet time to eat. Remind your body that you are no longer a teenager or a young adult. You have had lots of experience in curbing your cravings, and this case is not an exception.

Heartburn, Bloating, and Constipation

Occasionally, heartburn can occur when your stomach produces acids for digestion of your food, but there is no food present in the stomach to be digested. Bloating and constipation usually go hand in hand and can also occur in some cases. Together, these two can make you feel very uncomfortable.

Drinking adequate amounts of water can reduce the risk of heartburn, bloating, and constipation. Heartburns can also be minimized by cutting down on spicy foods during your eating window. If you experience heartburn during intermittent fasting, here's something you can try before going to sleep. Prop yourself up when you lie down to sleep. But don't use pillows to prop yourself as that will put more pressure on your stomach and increase the discomfort. Use a specially designed wedge or use a 6-inch block or something similar to elevate your head as you lie down. Doing this will make gravity minimize the backward flow of your stomach contents into your gullet. Propping yourself this way should bring you relief from heartburn. However, if heartburn, bloating, and constipation persist, consult your doctor immediately.

Binging

Eating a large amount as soon as the fasting window is over is usually associated with first-timers to fasting. The intense hunger of fasting can drive you to eat in a hurry when breaking, and you can end up overeating. In some cases, binging can be a result of a simple misunderstanding of the basics of intermittent fasting. They assume that they can eat as much as they want in the eating window since the no-eating window will take care of calories. This misunderstanding can deprive you of gaining any significant benefits that come with fasting intermittently, especially if you are looking to shed some weight. Binging or overeating in your eating window will reverse all the hard work you put in during the fast.

To avoid binging, ensure that the size and type of meal are planned well ahead of the eating window. Don't start fasting without knowing what portion you are going to consume at the end. Waiting until you can eat to decide what to eat and how much to eat can lead to overeating because your food choices will be largely influenced by how hungry you feel.

Low Energy

Feeling exhausted is a normal part of fasting. Until your body gets used to sourcing its fuel from fat storage, you are likely to experience some decline in your energy levels. Usually, they get back up within a couple of days.

To help stay energized, tailor your activities to remain low-key, at least at first. There is no need to push yourself to prove that you are a strong woman. Deciding to practice intermittent fasting is enough proof that you are mentally, emotionally, and physically strong. Since you are not in competition with anyone, it is in your best interest to conserve energy as much as possible. Get a massage, spend time relaxing in bed, or sleeping in if you have to.

Feeling Cold

Some people experience an extra feeling of cold during fasting. If you experience this, there is no cause for alarm. It might be a result of the drop in your blood sugar level. Usually, blood flow to your internal fat storage is increased during fasting. As a result of this increase, your fat is moved to parts of your body where it needs to be used as energy. This can make other parts of your body that have less fat storage experience cold. So if you feel cold in your fingers or toes, it is your body doing its fat burning process for your good.

To help reduce the cold, put on layers, stay in warm places, drink hot coffee or tea (with no calories), or take a hot shower. So avoid the urge to self-medicate. If the cold feeling persists even in your non-fasting days or in your eating window, consult your doctor.

Mood Swing

Imagine the following combinations. Stress on your body caused by the dip in your blood sugar. Your hormones are going berserk from the various reactions going on in your body as a result of not eating normally, or on schedule. The lethargic feeling from lack of food, hunger, and cravings constantly telling you to eat. Not being able to socialize with others freely because of the new eating pattern you can't wine and dine at social events if it is outside your eating window! All of these can lead to a psychological state of feeling annoyed or irritated.

The surest way to minimize mood swings resulting from intermittent fasting is to deliberately keep your attention off issues that set you on edge and focus on what you are doing and what makes you happy. The more you keep your mind wrapped up in gratitude and appreciation, the better you will feel. So, during your fasting window, be deliberate about engaging in things that lift your spirits and keep your mind on happy and productive thoughts.

Bottom Line

Intermittent fasting is a lifestyle regimen that is safe for older practitioners. It is a medical intervention that can bring about improvements in many aspects of a woman's health. However, it is not suitable for every person. If you notice that you have severe negative reactions to intermittent fasting, it is in your best interest to desist at once and consult your doctor. No rule makes it compulsory to complete a fast once you begin. You can break in the middle of your fasting window (even if it is just that day) if you can no longer endure unpleasant side effects and try again at a later time.

While it is okay to give your body a few weeks to get used to your new eating pattern, it is also crucial to pay close attention to what your body is telling you. Thankfully, as an older woman with experience, you can tell when something works for you or not. You know when you can commit to something and when you can't find the motivation to follow through. I believe that, as a woman with a tremendous wealth of experience, you will find the strength to stick to your resolve within reason.

CHAPTER 25:

Differences Between
the Young vs. Older Woman

At the most basic level, it must be said that there are detailed bodily differences between young women and older women. Many of these bodily differences become obvious with the outward, physical effects of aging, but a lot of them also happen on the inside, away from what our eyes can see.

When women age, enter and exit menopause, and become fully mature, their bodies change, reflecting different nutritional needs for the next 30+ years. During menopause, in particular, certain foods help with the urges, hot flashes, and more, but the period of intense transition is more of a gateway into a completely altered future (mentally, bodily, nutritionally, and more).

Women of this age experience slowed metabolism (to their great frustrations) as well as lowered hormone production. For weight and mood, therefore, menopause and maturation are equal disasters. Your body will go completely "out of whack," compared to how it used to function. You'll likely put on weight despite the dietary choices you make, and you may feel there's no relief in sight. Don't be fooled, however! Things may have changed for you, but they won't be stagnant changes.

Essentially, women at the stage of menopause and beyond need to absorb less energy overall from their food, yet they need more protein to deal with the effects of aging. Vitamins B12 & D, calcium, and zinc will need to be boosted, while the iron becomes less important for the aging female body. Vitamins C, E, A, & beta-carotene need to be increased too to fight off cancer, infection, disease, and more.

As the woman ages and matures even further, more things will change; mainly, she cannot bypass taking these important supplements any longer. In older and more mature women, the body's abilities to recognize hunger and thirst become muted, and dehydration poses a greater threat. Fewer calories are required for the older and more mature woman too, but she still needs to get as many nutrients as (if not more than!) the young woman does.

It seems that a younger woman can eat (relatively) what she wants and not worry about taking vitamins or supplements, but it is undeniable that the older woman will need this nutritional help to ensure longevity. Basically, health needs become more pressing for women at this age, as their bodies are less flexible and resistant to problems that may arise.

How IF Affects Women at This Age & How to Approach It

Because health, diet, reproductivity, and nutritional needs are all altered for mature and menopausal women, their relationships with intermittent fasting can be very different from young women's. For instance, while young women ought to be careful about how intermittent fasting can affect their fertility levels, older women can practice intermittent fasting freely without these concerns. Therefore, more mature women can apply the weight-loss techniques of intermittent fasting to their lives (and waistlines) without the worry of what negative side-effects might arise in the future.

For menopausal women, however, the situation is a little bit different than it is for fully mature women. People going through menopause have to deal with daily hormone fluctuations that cause hot and cold flashes, sleeplessness, anxiety, irregular periods, and more. At the beginning of this process, intermittent fasting will not necessarily help, and it could even make your situation more stressful.

For women in this situation who are actively going through menopause, you must remember that your body is extremely sensitive to changes right now. If you do find that intermittent fasting helps and that short periods of fast are effective, you must also make sure to increase the intensity of your fast as gradually as possible so your body can adjust without creating horrible hormonal repercussions for yourself and everyone around you. For the fully mature woman, intermittent fasting will not make you as cranky, moody, and irregular in the period, or otherwise because those hormones won't be affecting you at all anymore, or at least, hardly at all. Your dietary and eating schedule choices become more liberated from the effects they used to have on your hormonal health as the years go by. Therefore, if you're seeking weight loss, better energy, a physiological jolt back to health, or what have you, try out IF without concern and see what happens. For these types of women, intermittent fasting is set to provide hope through eased depression, the lessened likelihood of cancer (or its recurrence), promised weight loss, and more.

CHAPTER 26:

Difference Between Intermittent Fasting For Men And Women

Intermittent fasting is an effective lifestyle. It has proved to be a wondrous process for many people. Many people including men and women swear by intermittent fasting since it is the next best thing that has happened to them. Some are regularly sharing their success stories since intermittent fasting is quite an amazing process.

However, intermittent fasting is a very different process for men and women. Quite possibly intermittent fasting didn't work out for you or it is not producing the desired effect for you. There are a lot of things that need to be considered regarding this. I intend to cover all of them one by one.

The first thing that you should consider is that females have a body that is more complicated than men. For women above fifty, intermittent fasting doesn't generally lead to problems. A safer and controlled approach is always preferred.

However, some aged women swear the intermittent fasting messed up with their menopause or instead produced the opposite of what was desired. There are multiple reasons for that. The chief reason among them is some women try too hard or get their lessons from men coaches.

The first major difference between the bodies of men and women is the presence of different hormones. This is the reason why intermittent fasting is often a very different process for both genders. Here, I am talking about aged women and aged men. For some women, intermittent fasting can lead to a reduction of energy. When that happens, the women have increased sensitivity. This increased sensitivity can tell the body that it is not the time for hormones related to ovaries and fertility. Although in women above fifty, fertility is not a general problem, it can still lead to the shrinking of ovaries. This is a problem face specifically by women and not men. Therefore, unusual skipping of a meal can cause more harm than good since females have bodies that are more regulated to meal timings and calorie consumption than men.

The women have a protein present in them that is more sensitive to fasting than men. This protein alone is responsible for any changes that come due to fasting. The hormonal shift occurs due to the presence of this protein. This hormonal shift can easily affect the metabolism. Furthermore, it can seriously mess up your routine. As a woman above fifty, the change in metabolism can be hard to deal with.

In some of the cases for aged women, the nervous system was reported to have been negatively affected. In the case of men, intermittent fasting had provided a more relieving and calm sensation, reducing agitation. In the case of some women, the case was exactly the opposite. The nervous system became more agitated easily raising the irritability along with random mood swings. This is again linked to the body going into starvation. The main problem here is that in some cases, the body may require more nutrients than before. When menopause ends, some females may have a body that requires more calories for sustenance. Intermittent fasting may disrupt their calorie intake. In the case of men, such a scenario never occurs.

In some cases, although very limited research is involved, females have been reported to be affected adversely by intermittent fasting. The glucose tolerance was adversely affected.

The next difference is very encouraging. In the case of men, intermittent fasting does take effect and it affects them in a very similar manner to that of women. It gives them cholesterol reduction that leads to better resistance against heart diseases. However, in the case of women, the cholesterol reduction is more than that of men. Similarly, the increase in resistance against heart disease is also more than that of men. It is again linked to the enhanced sensitivity of women to intermittent fasting. This can be related to why some women have generally better results with intermittent fasting. For women who are suffering from diabetes or irregular periods, intermittent fasting can have a very negative effect. This is true for females who had a history of eating disorders.

CHAPTER 27:

Diet in Menopause

Menopause is one of the most complicated phases in a woman's life. The time when our bodies begin to change and important natural transitions occur that are too often negatively affected, while it is important to learn how to change our eating habits and eating patterns appropriately. It often happens that a woman is not ready for this new condition and experiences it with a feeling of defeat as an inevitable sign of time travel, and this feeling of prostration turns out to be too invasive and involves many aspects of one's stomach.

It is, therefore, important to remain calm as soon as there are messages about the first signs of change in our human body, to ward off the onset of menopause for the right purpose, and to minimize the negative effects of suffering, especially in the early days. Even during this difficult transition, targeted nutrition can be very beneficial.

What Happens to The Body of a Menopausal Woman?

It must be said that a balanced diet has been carried out in life and there are no major weight fluctuations, this will no doubt be a factor that supports women who are going through menopause, but that it is not a sufficient condition to present with classic symptoms that are felt, which can be classified according to the period experienced. In fact, we can distinguish between the pre-menopausal phase, which lasts around 45 to 50 years, and is physiologically compatible with a drastic reduction in the production of the hormone estrogen (responsible for the menstrual cycle, which starts irregularly.) This period is accompanied by a series of complex and highly subjective endocrine changes. Compare effectively: headache, depression, anxiety, and sleep disorders.

When someone enters actual menopause, estrogen hormone production decreases even more dramatically, the range of the symptoms widens, leading to large amounts of the hormone, for example, to a certain class called catecholamine adrenaline. The result of these changes is a dangerous heat wave, increased sweating, and the presence of tachycardia, which can be more or less severe.

However, the changes also affect the female genital organs, with the volume of the breasts, uterus, and ovaries decreasing. The mucous membranes become less active and vaginal dryness increases. There may also be changes in bone balance, with decreased calcium intake and increased mobilization at the expense of the skeletal system. Because of this, there is a lack of continuous bone formation, and conversely, erosion begins, which is a predisposition for osteoporosis.

Although menopause causes major changes that greatly change a woman's body and soul, metabolism is one of the worst. In fact, during menopause, the absorption and accumulation of sugars and triglycerides change and it is easy to increase some clinical values such as cholesterol and triglycerides, which lead to high blood pressure or arteriosclerosis. Also, many women often complain of disturbing circulatory disorders and local edema, especially in the stomach. It also makes weight gain easier, even though you haven't changed your eating habits.

The Ideal Diet for Menopause

In cases where disorders related to the arrival of menopause become difficult to manage, drug or natural therapy under medical supervision may be necessary. The contribution given by a correct diet at this time can be considerable, in fact, given the profound variables that come into play, it is necessary to modify our food routine, both in order not to be surprised by all these changes and to adapt in the most natural way possible.

The problem of fat accumulation in the abdominal area is always caused by the drop in estrogen. In fact, they are also responsible for the classic hourglass shape of most women, which consists of depositing fat mainly on the hips, which begins to fail with menopause. As a result, we go from a gynoid condition to an android one, with an adipose increase localized on the belly. Besides, the metabolic rate of disposal is reduced, this means that even if you do not change your diet and eat the same quantities of food as you always have, you could experience weight gain, which will be more marked in the presence of bad habits or irregular diet. The digestion is also slower and intestinal function becomes more complicated. This further contributes to swelling as well as the occurrence of intolerance and digestive disorders which have never been disturbed before. Therefore, the beginning will be more problematic and difficult to manage during this period. The distribution of nutrients must be different: reducing the amount of low carbohydrate, which is always preferred not to be purified, helps avoid the peak of insulin and at the same time maintains stable blood sugar.

Furthermore, it will be necessary to slightly increase the quantity of both animal and vegetable proteins; choose good fats, preferring seeds and extra virgin olive oil, and severely limit saturated fatty acids (those of animal origin such as lard, lard, etc.). All this to try to increase the proportion of antioxidants taken, which will help to counteract the effect of free radicals, whose concentration begins to increase during this period. It will be necessary to prefer foods rich in phytoestrogens, which will help to control the states of stress to which the body is subjected, and which will favor, at least in part, the overall estrogenic balance.

These molecules are divided into three main groups and the foods that contain them should never be missing on our tables: isoflavones, present mainly in legumes such as soy and red clover; lignans, of which flax seeds and oily seeds in general, are particularly rich; coumestans, found in sunflower seeds, beans, and sprouts. A calcium supplementation will be necessary through cheeses such as parmesan; dairy products such as yogurt, egg yolk, some vegetables such as rocket, Brussels sprouts, broccoli, spinach, asparagus; legumes; dried fruit such as nuts, almonds, or dried grapes.

Excellent additional habits that will help to regain well-being may be: limiting sweets to sporadic occasions, thus drastically reducing sugars (for example by giving up sugar in coffee and getting used to drinking it bitterly); learn how to dose alcohol a lot (avoiding spirits, liqueurs, and aperitif drinks) and choose only one glass of good wine when you are in company, this because it tends to increase visceral fat which is precisely what is going to settle at the level abdominal. Clearly, even by eating lots of fruit, it is difficult to reach a high carbohydrate quota as in a traditional diet. However, a dietary plan to follow can be useful to have a more precise indication of how to distribute the foods. One's diet must be structured in a personal way, based on specific metabolic needs and one's lifestyle.

CHAPTER 28:

Myths on Intermittent Fasting

Myth #1: Fasting is the Same as Starvation

When many people think about fasting, they think about starvation. After all, if you're not eating, then you must be starving. However, this myth isn't true. We fast every day, for about eight hours as we sleep, and yet we don't starve. You can even skip a meal on top of your sleep time, and not starve. Beyond just this basic daily fast we all do, starvation changes our body differently in comparison to intermittent fasting.

In the U.S. starvation is uncommon, though it's more common to have some food insecurity. If you are experiencing starvation, you'll have not eaten for a while, or eaten very low-calorie meals for several days. In fact, your starvation response starts after merely three days of not eating enough calories (Berg, Tymoczko, & Strye, 2002). During this time, you will lose weight, but you will also damage your body. In this case, your body and your brain know that you're starving, and they decide to try and save you. So your brain slows down your metabolism and sends out hormones to make you very hungry. Your body starts looking for food elsewhere. Now the science behind starvation is detailed, but suffice it to say, normally our body gets its energy from our food, which increases our blood-glucose levels, and our insulin— all of which feeds our body. However, when starving, our body runs out of its stores of glucose and starts searching for other sources of energy. In the search for protein, your body will start cannibalizing itself, eating through important cells, and muscles. It's not a quick process, because your body still needs to function to find more food.

However, without food, your body will slowly lose its functionality, leading to death.

Most of us won't starve to death in the U.S. Even when eating a very low-calorie diet, our body will keep pushing us to eat and with a lot of access to food, even if most is unhealthy, we're not likely to starve to death. However, we can still feel the effects of the starvation response without the right nutrition during the day. Not only will our brain keep sending out hunger warnings, but we'll also have a shift in emotions and sometimes, cognitive function. Researchers during WWII studied starvation to determine how our bodies react to it. This study is known as the Minnesota Starvation Experiment (Keys et al., 1950), and it found some interesting effects on our brains from starvation. Many of the participants experienced emotional swings, felt cognitively foggy, and had food dreams. They became depressed, anxious, and irritable. Physically, they experienced fluctuating body temperature, felt weak, and had reduced stamina. Their heart rate also decreased. These effects were felt in a stage of semi-starvation, where they were eating, but only a little every day, and very little of what they ate was healthy. So even when having food, we can experience the effects of starvation.

Intermittent fasting is very different from starvation because you won't be without food for three days. So long as you're following a set, healthy, fasting schedule, you will only be without food for 24 hours or less. So you will not initiate your natural starvation response. Our body is used to normal fasting, eating states. Once you eat your last meal before a fast, your body has high blood sugar levels, and increased insulin which are all fueling your body. The body also stores the extra glucose and puts it aside for later. After the first several hours, your body starts to reduce its insulin levels and your blood sugar levels also drop. Your liver releases its stores of glucose and then your body starts using fatty tissue to continue fueling itself since its blood-sugar levels are lower. This state is known as ketosis. Your body remains in this state for a while, even when you eat again (Berg, Tymoczko, & Strye, 2002). Because you're providing your body with food, even after 24 hours without, your body doesn't shift into its starvation response. Instead, it sticks with its stage of ketosis, with reduced insulin levels and blood-sugar levels, before getting more energy from your next meal.

It's important to note that while there are differences between starvation and fasting, any fast taken for too long will result in starvation. Any diet, where you are eating less than 1000 calories a day, puts you at risk for starting your body's starvation response. However, this response won't happen immediately. So long as you are eating something during your days, you'll be ok. In most fasts, you're going to eat your regular daily calories every day. But in some fasts like the 5/2 and the Alternate Day fasting, you'll have periods of low-calorie intake. Even during these periods, you'll only be without food for 24 hours or less. So, while doing intermittent fasting, your body shouldn't have a starvation response.

Myth #2: Fasting will Make You Gain Weight

This myth is closely related to the previous myth. It's connected to the starvation response, or as many people call it, "Starvation Mode." Starvation mode is the same thing as our starvation response, but just in a more sensationalized perspective. The general myth most people have is that fasting will put you into starvation mode, which means your metabolism slows down, you'll start hoarding all the fuel your body takes in because of the slow metabolism, and thus, you'll gain weight. Let's break this down because it's a complicated myth.

We've already covered how fasting won't put you into starvation mode if it's done correctly. So we're going to explore the metabolism aspect. When you're starving, and your body/brain starts trying to save itself, it starts to lower its metabolism. Your metabolism is what helps you maintain your body's weight and repair your cells. It's how your body processes the food you eat and turns it into the fuel used to power your every action. During starvation, your metabolism rate will reduce because you don't have enough food to keep it running at its optimal level. This is to conserve energy for your most important living functions. Because people often think that fasting is the same as starvation, they expect your metabolism to slow while fasting, resulting in you gaining weight. This is confusing because during starvation, yes, your metabolic rate decreases, but your body is using all the stores it has. This means that there isn't any extra fuel! You will not gain weight when you're starving. It's impossible. So, carrying that belief over to fasting just doesn't work.

In most diet cultures, you'll hear people talk about "fast" metabolism and "slow" metabolism. Having a fast metabolism is supposed to help you lose weight because you're burning more food and fuel than you're eating and storing. Slow metabolism is supposed to make you gain weight because you're not burning enough fuel and everything extra you eat gets stored. So when people think about this myth, they think that your lack of food will reduce your metabolism, which will lead to more food storage, with less energy and stores being used. However, this isn't true with fasting. Fasting improves your metabolism and uses your stores of energy efficiently (Patterson et al., 2016). Done right, you will likely lose weight when fasting, not gain weight.

While I'd like to fully debunk this myth, there is some truth to it, and it all comes down to diet. It's possible that you can gain weight when fasting, but it's not because of your metabolic rate. If you choose to eat regular meals that exceed your daily calories, then you're going to gain weight. This is the same with any diet, any fast, or any food you eat. If you exceed what your body will use, energy/food-wise, then you'll gain weight. So, you may gain weight when fasting. But if you do, it's not because of a lower metabolic rate and is more because of a poorly planned diet. To prevent this, you must eat well-balanced nutritious foods. This will help you maintain weight, or possibly lose some if it's a shift from your normal diet. Basically, if you gain weight when fasting, then it's due to diet and you'll need to watch what you eat to lose or maintain your weight.

Myth #3: Fasting is not Sustainable Long-term

There are so many diets out there that are not sustainable. What immediately comes to mind are the types of diet where you eat only one type of food, like the cabbage soup diet. These kinds of diets are not sustainable because it's easy to start craving more types of food. Your body itself will crave the nutrients it needs, while you'll get bored with that single kind of food. A lot of diets that are fad diets aren't sustainable because they often don't provide your body with the requirements it needs to function well. This results in you being hungry and craving the foods that are prohibited in those diets. Fasting isn't like a fad and doesn't restrict certain types of food. So, while you might get hungry, it's unlikely you'll have any brutal cravings. This can increase the sustainability of fasting.

Also, there are so many kinds of fasting. Some of them are easy to incorporate into your daily life, like the 14/10 fast or the 16/8 fast. With these diets, you're simply extending your fast further than your normal eight hours of sleep. Sometimes this means eating your last meal early, or your first meal late. Because these two types are simple and easy to get into, they can be easy to maintain as well. Other types of fasting can be even easier, depending on your personality. But the reality remains that fasting can be quickly started and maintained.

Finally, a lot of people find fasting much easier to sustain than long-term calorie restriction. Long-term calorie restriction is your typical, doctor-approved diet. You reduce your eaten calories by a bit every day and you lose weight. However, this can be difficult to maintain because it requires you to pick and choose what you eat carefully and can restrict social eating. In a study comparing alternate-day fasting and calorie restriction, the researchers found that the participants felt the fasting was easier to sustain (Alhamdan, 2016). This has been echoed in other studies and even anecdotally. Even though hunger could be an issue with alternate-day fasting, that's not always the case as participants found that their hunger on fasting days was reduced after two weeks of following the fast schedule (Klemple et al., 2010). So, fasting can be easy to start, maintain, and sustain because it doesn't restrict you.

Intermittent fasting is considered a lifestyle change. I know this is mentioned in many different diets, but fasting, it's the easiest way to change your eating habits. It can change your health and reduce your weight. By following it in the long-term, you'll maintain all those benefits. So, fasting is and can be sustainable.

CHAPTER 29:

FAQs About Intermittent Fasting

How long will I continue to fast?

Did you know that there are many commonalities between this feeding system and how naturally slender people eat? Some days they eat other times they just miss meals, that's how the nutrition is. If you become familiar with your selected IF schedule, your calorie intake will decrease until it becomes normal for you. You can change your frequency once you get the weight you need. It's best to keep fasting and not stop at all. It aims to permanently change your lifestyle, not just for a short time. It is a daily practice that guarantees consistent weight reduction.

I take some medications which require me to eat, what do I do during the fasting times to take the medicine?

You can experience some side effects when you take any medicines on an empty belly. Iron supplements can cause sickness and nausea; aspirin can cause stomach ulcers and upsets. It's better to ask the doctor if you should take this drug as you continue a fast.

You can take the medicine with small, low-calorie leafy vegetables that do not interfere with your pace. Your blood pressure can drop over the fasting period so that if you take blood pressure-lowering medicine, the blood pressure may become too low and lead to headaches.

What food is better to eat raw or cooked vegetables?

There have been several discussions on this subject. Some argue that food preparation leads to vitamins, enzymes, and minerals destruction. But it also makes cellulose fiber more available for your system, among other nutrients. When prepared, carrots, fungi, spinach, chips, and other peppers, other vegetables provide more antioxidants, but the disadvantage is that Vitamin C may be lost when cooking. There is no official response; all you have to do is eat plenty of vegetables in whatever way you want.

I am old, is it too late for me to start fasting?

Starting fasting can never be too late. It can help you manage your appetite, help you lose weight, and even make your life longer. You'll quickly notice the impacts; you'll feel healthier, slimmer, and stronger. Start immediately.

When I take a treat like a packet of chips during my fasting period, what's going to happen?

Fasting is an intermittent activity involving voluntary meal abstinence. Not only does it help you, because you consume fewer calories, it's also because that's what your flesh was built to do. Do not equate fasting with starvation because starvation is bad, but fasting is good. IF's aim is to provide your body with free time to relax from food. Your improvement will end with just one snack and your blood sugar levels will allow you to get out of a fasted state.

What should I do if I don't lose weight?

Weight loss is a gradual process that takes quite some time to accomplish thus patients and consistency are needed. If you don't lose some weight in the first few weeks you should just keep going, you shouldn't be concerned. If you're going for an even longer period and still don't lose weight, it's wise to review what you eat as this is the most likely cause of the problems you might have. It's important to keep track of the food you eat so you can track the problem easily.

During my period, is it really safe to fast?

Fasting is not at all right when you are pregnant or breastfeeding, but your monthly cycles will not affect your fast in any way unless they are very painful or intolerable. If so, you can test your iron levels and take supplements as well.

I have diabetes, can I still practice IF?

If you have type 1 or type 2 diabetes or on diabetes medication you need to take additional care while practicing IF. If the need arises, your doctor will check your blood sugar levels carefully to change your medicine prescription to allow them to co-exist with intermittent fasting peacefully. When you can't be closely monitored, don't attempt fasting. It decreases the blood sugar levels and continuing to take drugs as insulin can lead to exceptionally low concentrations of blood glucose that lead to hypoglycemia. You can drink a sugar-filled drink like soda and even stay off your fasting routine one day to raise the level of blood sugar. If you have blood sugar levels that are excessively low, this is due to over-medication and not intermittent fasting. Reduce your use of medications in advance because you expect lower levels of blood sugar when you begin IF.

Is it true that I can eat all I want on non-fast days?

This is true as all foods are allowed. It is permissible to use anything from the most oil-drenched fried chicken to a vegetable salad for any other meat. It is best not to consume too much as if during the time you were fasting you are struggling to eat what you would have. You may even overcome the impacts of fasting when you overfeed. It should not be made into a ritual of overeating after fasting, eating should be done responsibly. But it all boils down to what you want to do as you are the one that decides to fast and by now you already know a lot of the do and don't. You'll automatically find yourself choosing healthier meals after doing the fasting for some time.

Can I get tired from fasting, if so, how could I stop it?

No, the opposite would happen. Individuals have more strength in fasting as a result of higher levels of adrenaline in the body. With more than enough energy, you will certainly be able to conduct your ordinary operations. Fatigue is not a normal part of fasting, so if you feel extremely exhausted, stop fasting right away and see a doctor right away.

Can I receive the same benefits of fasting as an adult of the opposite sex?

Hormonally and metabolically, there are several differences between men and women. For example, women store more fat and are more susceptible to exercise-dependent fat burning. Research has shown that fasting females respond more quickly to endurance exercise while fasting males react more quickly with a weighted workout. IF's benefits on both genders are almost equal. It's not supposed to be a race, but more of an individual experience, so concentrating on your body is better than thinking about others.

During the first days of fasting, I want to use meal replacement shakes, is it all right or should I just stick to food?

During the first days of IF training, these meal replacement shakes have helped most individuals. These are definitely better than calorie counting, as you can just sip free from your thirst. Even if the real nutrition is considered to be more effective when you like these drinks, you can go ahead and use them. Make sure that you only have those that have small or even no glucose.

Can I get the intermittent fasting result in me getting headaches?

Sure, but it only happens due to fatigue and not due to inadequate calories.

You may have withdrawal symptoms, but they are gentle. Make sure you take medication on an ongoing basis to treat the migraine as you would a normal one. If during the fasting period you feel ill you must stop immediately.

If I observe intermittent fasting, what amount of weight can I lose?

That's based on many factors and variations between individuals. Such factors are your heart rate, your exercise level, and how closely you observe the pace.

During the first week, you will lose water and you will eventually lose weight as a result of your daily calorie intake. It's not advised to lose really fast weight and shouldn't be an aim, it's better to lose a little weight continuously.

Could I easily get cranky as I practice IF?

It has been used in all hundreds of years; this has never been an issue; it is not even in societies that have fasting as an essential part of their beliefs. Moreover, Buddhist monks are considered to be very peaceful people while they practically fast daily, fasting has no such effect.

I happen to be naturally slender thus I don't require any weight loss, can still practice IF for its physiological benefits?

If you're comfortable with your weight that's fine, fasting is very much still an option you have to improve your health. You have to make sure that during your feeding time you focus more on calorie-dense meals. Most slender people who fast get all the advantages without any problem. Testing through trial and error is the only way you can find the right balance between eating and fasting to keep you at a safe weight. Reduce the days of fasting by constantly checking your weight and take care not to get underweight as that would be hazardous to you.

Can I get too much food as a result of fasting?

The answer is yes and no to this question. First, it's really because you're going to consume more than you usually do after fasting. It is not, however, since feeding above the regular amounts in no days of fasting is not a consequence of fasting.

I'm going to sleep hungry when my fasting time is at night?

It's not probable, but it's mainly dependent on your metabolism, just try to keep your mind away from food and feel hungry. When you get out of your bed you may not feel hungry at all. Essentially, your appetite and hunger will suit your fasting routine.

Can IF make my body go into starvation mode to prevent more loss of fat?

This is not a realistic side effect because there is no calorie restriction on IF. There's no IF routine that's intense to the point you're going into starvation mode. The fasting time is short, so from the fat stores, the body absorbs fat and retains muscle mass. Research has shown that IF does not lower any individual's metabolic rate. Despite long fasts like those for three days, there will be no decrease in the basal metabolic rate. There is also no increase in the hunger hormone called ghrelin during IF.

I'm an overweight fellow, is IF really the key to solving my problem?

Intermittent fasting has proved to be one of the most effective and enduring strategies for obese individuals to lose and retain new weight. The bigger you are, the greater the initial loss of weight. You've most likely given up conventional restrictive diets. Intermittent fasting has an advantage over all of them because it is more versatile and when you consume anything it is not a crime because nothing is restricted. Research has shown that obese individuals are very easily used to fasting.

Can I eat during my fasting time if I really have to like during celebrations and major ceremonies?

Be active, but concentrate on what you're ingesting. While it's vital to get help from your family and friends, if you keep telling them you can't eat as you are in a fast, they'll start to get tired of hearing that, and eventually, you'll feel self-conscious. This will render it an obstacle to your normal activity, which is not its original intent, rather than something that fits perfectly in your life. When you know that there is a social event connected to food, then fast the day before or the day before. It is a very flexible device and without any difficulties, you will continue to be active and enjoy these times.

CHAPTER 30:

How To Manage Hunger Attacks

I wish I could tell you that fasting is all sunshine and roses. I wish I could tell you that it's so easy to follow. Unfortunately, it's not. There are going to be days when you look at your cup of coffee and cry because you can't eat anything for another four hours. There are going to be days when you throw yourself at the doors of the local cafe and ogle all the pastries and lattes, knowing that by the time you can eat, the doors will be closed. There will be days when all your friends are out drinking and partying, and you're eating window just ended. Basically, there are going to be frustrating days, sad days, difficult days, stressful days, and nightmare days where you're going to want to throw in the towel and give up on your fast. These are the kinds of days that you'll need the motivation to help you continue your fast. Without the motivation, you'll likely end your fasting period early, not start the next fasting period, or just give up altogether. One key thing you can do to keep yourself motivated is to remind yourself of the amazing days. Think about that day last week, when you had your latte and your boss didn't yell at you. Think about that morning, when your dog lovingly jumped on the bed and woke you up with millions of kisses. Think about that time that you dropped your scarf on the train and someone found it and returned it to you. The recollection of these good days can help remind you that your days will get better. You can use these reminders on the rough days when you just want to give up on fasting, or the days when you just want to sit on the bathroom floor and cry. When your days are rough and you have the stress of fasting on top of that, you'll likely break your fast. However, you must continue your fast again in the future, even if you hit some speed bumps along the way.

Distract Yourself

Sometimes the hunger that comes with fasting can be overwhelming. This is especially true with fasts that require 24 hours of not eating. If you can't seem to stop thinking about food, or if you're just feeling gnawing hunger, then you might want to break your fast early and just eat everything in front of you. Before doing that, see if some distractions will help you maintain your fasts. Some good distractions include work, exercise, and meditation.

Work probably shouldn't be classified as a distraction, but it can be a useful one when you're fasting. Having your mind occupied by something that requires you to be actively engaged is a great way to distract yourself from your feelings of hunger. Many of us have already experienced this. If you've ever been in the 'flow' while working, you've probably skipped meals without realizing it. You may have even come out of the flow and realized that hours have gone by and your stomach is growling at you. This realization can help you when you're fasting. You can try to get into a state of flow, but if that is beyond you at that moment, then just get engaged with work. Start a new project or plan. If your work is very active, then get fully engaged with the activity. If your work is passive, then find another way to distract yourself.

One way of distracting yourself is to do some light exercises. Depending on the fast you're following, heavy exercise might be too much. Light exercises, on the other hand, can be a great distraction and won't affect you negatively. Light exercises include things like walking and yoga. They aren't high intensity and don't involve too much effort on your part. So, they shouldn't cause you to feel nauseous or faint. Walking outside in nature is a perfect distraction. Instead of walking and focusing on your hunger, focus on things outside of you. Look at the trees, birds, and insects. Observe the other people around you, breathe in deeply, and just walk. Allow your mind to wander, but if it keeps going to your hunger, then refocus on something else. Yoga is another way that you can distract yourself. Because it requires more focus on the positions and your breath, you will quickly find yourself distracted from your hunger.

Use your distractions wisely. While it's okay to distract yourself from feeling hungry, it's not okay to distract yourself from feeling intensely uncomfortable. If you're feeling unwell, then this is a sign to step back from the fast and speak to a doctor. Don't "power through" something that isn't working for you.

Remind Yourself of Your Goals

When you fast, you usually have reasons for why you are choosing to do it. Maybe your goal is to lose weight, maybe it's just gone get healthier in general. Your goals should be personal to you, not something that's mimicry of other people's goals. Think about why you want to fast. Think about a goal that will motivate you to continue fasting. Whatever your reasoning, your goals can help you maintain motivation. To help you remember your goals, write them down. You can put them in the same journal you put your food notes in, or you can make a specific fasting journal with your fasting schedule, food notes, and goals altogether. Having them written down makes them more concrete and gives you something to look back on when your fast becomes difficult to sustain.

As you start to feel weary of continuing your fast, or if you struggle with the hours without food, then take the time to say your goals. Write them down somewhere so you see them frequently. You can use a dry erase marker and put your goals on your bathroom mirror. That way every day as you start your eating window you can see your goals, and every evening as you bring your eating window to a close, you're reminded of why you're fasting. During the day, when you struggle with your fast, take a moment to repeat your goals to yourself. You can say it like a mantra to help you stay focused and ignore the hunger.

Beyond repeating your goals to yourself, you can create a visual to help embody your goals. You can create a vision board. A lot of people create these boards to help remind them of their goals in many aspects of their lives. Usually, it's created with cutouts from magazines or printed pictures. Each image represents something specific to you. If your goal is to buy a house, then you might have a picture of a beautiful house. For fasting, if your goal is to be healthier, then your picture can be anything that embodies the word "health" to you. It could be people exercising, or even just a mountain with clean air. Your images are unique to you. Once you have your goal images, put them together in a collage and post them somewhere that you'll see your vision board every day. Your office or kitchen, maybe your bedroom, are all good choices.

Finally, if fasting is getting you down and you don't have your vision board or written goals near at hand, then do a visualization technique. Close your eyes and in your mind, visualize yourself as you have reached your goal. What do you look like? What emotions do you feel? How do you feel physically? How do you feel mentally? Consider all these questions to help you visualize your goal achievement. This can help you remain motivated to fasting, and encourage you to keep going, even after you've broken your fast.

Be Compassionate Towards Yourself

Have you ever notices that the closer we are to someone, the harsher we are to them? Like, our acquaintances see us as these perfect angels, but our friends know that we have a sharp wit and an even sharper tongue. Our family knows that we don't take any nonsense from anyone and our family gets the big brunt of our anger when we feel miserable. But the person we treat the worst is ourselves. Any slight failure or disillusionment results in us reprimanding ourselves. Comments like, "I'm so stupid" or "Why am I such an idiot?" are things that we say to ourselves. We would never say them to our friends or acquaintances. So, we're insanely harsh to ourselves.

When to hit a snag with fasting, maybe cheat a little with what we eat, or skip a fasting period, it's not uncommon for us to have some self-recriminating thoughts. These thoughts aren't beneficial. They often tear us down without providing an area to build ourselves up again. They can be extremely negative and result in us giving up our fasts altogether. Instead of sulking with our thoughts and giving up on our fasts, we should try to practice a little self-kindness.

What would you say to a friend who said they failed at their fast and they're so stupid? Would you agree with them? That's unlikely. It's more likely that you'll try to console them, reassure them that they aren't stupid, and follow up by encouraging them to continue trying. Do the same thing that you would do for a friend but do it for yourself. Instead of saying, "I'm so stupid, I failed," say, "I took a cheat day, and that's okay. I'll get right back into my fasting schedule." Be positive and compassionate towards yourself. We all make mistakes and we all have lapses. Simply learn from your experience, adapt your fasting schedule to accommodate what you've learned, and start fasting again. Don't give up just because of a little bump in the road.

Get Some Support + Bonus 16/8 method

Things are always easier with support. Some of us like to think that we're eagles, living solo among all the turkeys. We want to be free without anyone there to back us up. We don't need them! But this isn't ideal, especially when things are difficult. Sometimes, it's better to be surrounded by turkeys who care about you and will support you. Sometimes it's better to be the turkey because you know you're lovingly supported by your friends and family with you. What I'm trying to say here is that when you struggle with intermittent fasting, having the support of your friends can make a difference in your success or failure.

If you have some friends who are very supportive of you, make sure they know when you're struggling with your fasting goals. They can probably give you a good shoulder to cry on and may even give you some tips for how to make things easier. If you're very lucky, your friends may join your fast with you. This way, you can keep each other accountable. If they don't want to fast, that's okay too so long as they're supportive of you following your health goals.

If you're truly an eagle, alone in the world, then seek support from online communities. There are a lot of blogs and forums out there, dedicated to intermittent fasting. Join some of them and talk to others who are struggling. Some great forums to join include the Reddit forum on intermittent fasting. There, they post pictures of success, questions about speed bumps, and even give each other motivation. Get involved and you'll have some support too.

In conclusion, fasting is hard, but it can be done with the right support behind you and the motivation to push forward. Keep persevering, keep trying, and only give up if your body can't handle the fast. Even when you make a mistake or take a cheat day (or month), just try again when you're ready. Keep trying.

CHAPTER 31:

Exercises that Can Help to Lose Weight After 50

To understand the science of intermittent fasting, the basics of nutrition need to be looked into. And it's pretty straightforward: the food we eat is broken down into molecules and ends up in our blood that feeds our bodies' cells. Net carbohydrates (all carbs in the meal minus the fiber) are part of those molecules, and our body turns them into sugar (glucose), so our cells could use them for energy. To be able to use sugar for power, we need insulin, which is produced in our pancreas every time we throw carbohydrates into some food. Any excess sugar we don't eat gets stored in the form of fat with the expectation that we'll use that fat for energy later, once we've got no sugar left. The right way to NOT end up with vast stores of fat (and become overweight) is to spend the same amount of energy you get from the food. Life, however, isn't perfect, and many of us have habits that restrict our chances of moving all day long. Office workers tend to sit 75 % of their waking hours. So, what should we do to lose weight or not gain weight?

One way to do this is to focus on increasing your energy consumption by increasing physical activity or in terms of a layman–exercising and doing sport. But you already knew that one, right? Another approach, though, is to concentrate on consuming less food than you need for the energy that day, generating a caloric deficit as a result. And this is where intermittent fasting enters.

Intermittent fasting facilitates the reduction of the number of meals and calories you eat per day. For some time, it is much more convenient not to eat at all vs. eating less Restricting meal frequency ends up reducing insulin to low enough levels and long enough to get our bodies into ketosis mode–a magical state where we use fat for energy vs. sugar. And as a result, you are losing weight. But please be careful-it will only be beneficial to reduce the number of meals or the number of hours you eat per day if you consume fewer calories than you need.

The good news, right? You can altogether avoid metabolic syndrome, and "it's never too late to start exercising," we have middle-aged people going to the gym who have never worked out and rowing a half-marathon within four months. Exercising is even more successful when paired with a healthy diet. There are some obstacles to get your exercise groove on after age 50: women experience age-related declines.

1. Walking:

Not only is it a great way to lose weight because you don't need to be part of a gym or invest in special equipment, but it's also a perfect workout for older adults because it's gentle on your joints and helps to keep your heart and bones healthy. While walking at a slow pace (3.5 mph) for half an hour, a 155-pound person consumes 149 calories, raises the speed to 4 mph, and the same person burns 167calories.

Of course, running burns calories at the same time, but walking is an approachable, low-impact exercise that works for the majority. (Bonus points for exercising in nature: free-spending time has a lot of physical, social, and emotional benefits.) For regular weight loss, you'll need to watch at least twenty minutes of brisk walking most days of the week.

2. Lifting Weights:

It not only helps you burn fat, but also improves your ability to perform daily tasks such as carrying grocery stores, climbing stairs, and other household tasks. Lifting weights is critical because each year, we all lose 1% or 2 % of our muscle strength. Free weight resistance training is crucial to weight loss; plus, right leg and hip muscles reduce your risk of falling, which is a significant cause of impairment in older adults.

Montoya recommends strength training at least twice a week for the lifting of newbies, with workouts being divided between upper-body exercises one day and lower-body exercises the other.

Tip: Skip the resistance machines and keep increasing your lifting weight as soon as it gets quick.

Older people tend to use only resistance machines, but I prefer using free weights because they require strength, and they enable more joint stabilizer muscle activity.

3. Yoga:

Not only does yoga make your muscles stronger, but it also increases your flexibility. Another advantage: during yoga, stretching and breathing deeply helps to reduce stress hormones that contribute to belly fat, a common problem for anyone over 50 years old. And since yoga lowers levels of stress, it also has the potential to improve your overall eating habits (less stress eating!), thus promoting weight loss.

Indeed, a study shows men lost fat by committing to a 14-week yoga program. The study people practiced 90 minutes of yoga five days a week, but don't worry, every little bit counts.

4. Interval Training:

If you're up for it, high-intensity interval training (HIIT), which is any workout where you alternate between intense activity and less intense activity, will help you burn more calories. It's one of the effective ways to lose weight, as long as you have permission from your doctor for strenuous exercise.

For older people, just starting the best HIIT activities include swimming and cycling. You will see significant improvements in your aerobic fitness, strength, and blood-pressure readings by doing somewhat hard intervals, followed by easy intervals.

For the best results, Montoya suggests these intervals: five minutes of brisk walking, followed by five minutes of casual walking, three minutes on, three minutes rest, one-minute rest, one-minute rest, and repeat. One can find the same pattern on the bike or in the pool. Start three days a week with a 30-minute workout period, and work up from there.

5. Build Lean Muscle Rapidly

Particularly in the weight room, patience is overrated, and especially when it comes to those concentrating on a particular outcome: muscle development.

Change takes time, of course, but if you're struggling to grow and build muscle, and don't see any noticeable increase in size from month to month, it's a sign your approach is off. And a workout is a dreadful thing to waste on. Plus, even if you see progress, there is no reason for you not to see more.

How do you revive your performance? There are seven ways here.

1. Increase Your Training Volume:

Training volume multiplied by your number of sets; your number of reps is a primary determinant of hypertrophy (aka how to grow muscle). And to increase volume, you might have to go down in weight than you might think.

Similar to strength training, the intensity will decrease during a program's hypertrophy process, with intensity sitting between 50 % and 75 % of the person's 1RM, the maximum weight he or she can lift for one rep. Do each of the lifts for three to six sets of 10 to 20 reps 2 to get the amount the muscles need.

2. Focus on the Eccentric Phase:

If you lift some weight, you have a concentrate (hard) and an eccentric phase (easy). For example, as you descend into a squat, you are performing a strange action. That is the focus when you return to standing. Yet the eccentric study is far stronger at causing hypertrophy, according to studies.

To maximize your workout's amount of eccentric effort, you can do two things: either slow down the strange process of each exercise you perform or incorporate unusual variations into your routine.

Take the squat, for example; you'd lower to the floor to make it eccentric-only, and end the exercise there. Note: If you're trying exercise-only, you'll need to increase the weight you're using substantially. Physiologically, muscles move eccentrically far stronger than they do concentrative.

3. Reduce Between-Set Rest Intervals:

If you are touching your phone between exercise sets, it is better to set the timer to 30 to 90 seconds. Rest periods of 30 to 90 seconds when lifting for hypertrophy encourage a rapid release into muscle-building hormones (including testosterone and human growth hormone) while also ensuring that you tire your muscles.

Research published last year suggests that fatigue of your muscles is a prerequisite for hypertrophy, regardless of the rep and set scheme. Don't get scared of feeling the pain.

4. Eat More Protein:

Training breaks down your muscles to grow muscle. Protein builds them up again. And the harder you lift workouts, the more important it is to consider protein intake to solidify recovery from the muscle-building foods.

For optimum protein growth, weight lifters need to eat 0.25 to 0.30 grams of protein per kilogram of body weight per meal, according to research from the University of Sterling. This works out to 20 to 24 grams of protein at each meal for a 175-pound male. You will get this in three to four eggs, a cup of Greek yogurt, or a protein scoop powder.

5. Focus on Calorie Surpluses, Not Deficits:

This can be hard to get used to, especially for those who are used to calorie counting in hopes of weight loss. But to build muscle mass most effectively quickly (meaning weight gained, not lost), you need to consume more calories than you burn every day.

That's because when your body feels it's in a calorie deficit because you're eating fewer calories than you're burning every day, it slows down the urge of your body to build new muscle. After all, if your body thinks that food is in short supply, having a sole won't be the prime concern.

Aim at eating around 250 to 500 extra calories per day. So ensure all weight gained comes from the muscle; the majority of those calories should come from protein. In a study conducted by the Pennington Biomedical Research Center in 2014, people who ate a high-calorie protein-rich diet stored about 45 percent of those calories as muscle, while those who followed a low-protein diet with the same number of calories stored 95 % as fat.

6. Snack on Casein Before Bed:

Long common among bodybuilders, casein protein gradually absorbs into the bloodstream, ensuring that it keeps the muscles filled with amino acids longer than other protein forms such as whey and plant proteins. In one study of Medicine and Science in Sports and Exercise, consuming casein protein immediately before bed boosted the circulating amino acid levels of young men for 7.5 hours; they built muscle throughout the night while they were sleeping.

Try cottage cheese, Greek yogurt, and milk, to get some pre-bed casein. The casein-based protein powder works like a charm for smoothie lovers.

7. Get More Sleep:

One needs more than the right nutrition to recover the muscle. Recovery time takes about eight hours per night. After all, the body releases human growth hormone as you sleep, which helps the tissue development and keeps the stress hormone cortisol levels in check.

Furthermore, a study shows that sleeping for five hours, as opposed to eight hours, reduces muscle-building testosterone levels by a whopping 10 % to 15 % every night for just one week.

The National Sleep Foundation suggests adults aged between 18 and 64 sleep seven to nine hours a night. No apologies.

CHAPTER 32:

Success Stories

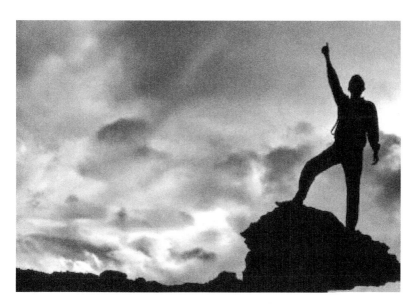

If you have any doubts, then look to those who have tread before you. These stories are from real women who have lost weight using IF. Most people who try this way of eating are very happy with their results. Some people are mad because they cannot lose weight rapidly or because they have no results because they eat mountains of food in their eating windows. The ones who do it right are inspirational successes.

Amanda's Fasting Story

"I'm not sure where I first heard about IF. Probably some celebrity-inspired me. Generally, I hate diets, and I would never have undergone this type of nutritional restriction. I believe in enjoying life and eating when you want to. But I had several health problems, including being overweight. I was thirty pounds overweight.

I read that you should go for 10 to 20 hours without eating. So, I chose to go 16 hours without eating as a nice middle ground. Thus, I eat at 5 pm and then go to bed and have breakfast at eight. Obviously, it worked for me.

But I will tell you what was so hard. The hard part was not eating a nighttime meal. I had to get over that and just sip hot chicory tea. That's a lifesaver, by the way. I love chicory tea. I miss milk, but I use tea and water to fill the 15-16 fasting hours. I keep myself busy and sleep like a baby. It helped me get over the need to snack before bed. Now I enjoy my meals so much more. They are not a routine or chore to fix, but a pleasure that I look forward to.

I loved how adjustable it is, too. One time I had a late office dinner. Easy enough, I just switched breakfast to be at 11 am. It works seamlessly with your schedule. Just keep on top of the hours, and you're good.

During my first month, I dropped ten pounds. Whoohoo! It showed right away. People kept giving me compliments. I didn't mean for these awesome results; they just happened. I didn't have any food restrictions, and I didn't hate my life. I just had to watch when I ate. That's all.

And, my stomach has decreased in inches. I fit in old dresses again! I eat smaller portions as a result. The minute I get full, I don't want to eat anymore. I eat in the morning, but I usually don't want to, I chew to get my calories. I have lost edema in most of my body, and my blood pressure is normal. I sleep better because of the chicory, too. I have no more constipation or stomach pain. I recommend this approach for everyone, and I think everyone should adhere to it as much as possible. It's a great program that works with your body."

Rose's Fasting Story

"By accident, I found out about the 16/8 fasting system, and I researched it thoroughly. I also asked friends and acquaintances. They had all loved it. So, I decided to try it out for myself and share what happened. So far, I've been doing this plan for three weeks. I have already lost ten pounds. I fast for 16 hours and then eat for eight hours. The fasting starts after I eat dinner and lasts for 16 hours until I have breakfast. Generally, I eat at 8 pm and then again at noon. I just adjust the times if I eat earlier or later. It is so simple; anyone can do it. I don't have tons of eating restrictions, but I do eat more protein now. For the 16 hours, my body just rests and cleanses.

At first, it was pretty difficult. I was taught that breakfast is the most important meal of the day, so I felt like I was committing some sin when I would go to work without breakfast in my belly. My whole life, I would eat a big breakfast of cereal, boiled eggs, sandwiches, and even a smoothie. Giving it up made me feel like something was wrong. For a few days, my schedule was all out-of-whack, and I was incredibly hungry by lunchtime. By the end of a week, though, that all passed. I began to feel lighter and not look at the clock waiting for noon.

You don't have to skip breakfast, by the way. That's just what I did. You can eat in the morning and eat dinner earlier. If you need your morning meal, do it. That's what is great about this system; you can make it work for you. I can honestly say that I don't miss breakfast much, though.

You don't have to give up the foods you love. You can still eat your favorite dessert! I love chocolate, so I eat that during my window. What diet allows you to do that? Uh, this one! But this plan isn't really a diet, just a power system. I feel light, and I'm losing fat, not muscle mass. Don't torture yourself with fad diets that don't work; use this power system and enjoy the results. IF is really just a simple lifestyle change you can fit into your daily life."

Ellice's Fasting Story

"I had pretty much given up on remission from rheumatoid arthritis after giving birth. I was on the verge of despair, both physically and mentally. My quality of life was so low. Drug treatments don't work well for me, and my family has a long history of Type 1 Diabetes. I knew that I would develop diabetes because of the sudden jumps my pancreas was doing. I knew that something was wrong because I would break out in cold sweats and then feel terrible weakness until I ate. I didn't know what to do, and my options seemed nonexistent.

But on some baby board, I found some women raving about IF. Well, why not try it? Nothing else was working.

I started experimenting with it. It wasn't so bad. I have started going longer times with my fasts. Recently, I made it 36 hours! I noticed that after starting this practice, I felt way better in the mornings. Usually, I hurt the worst in my joints at this time, so the pain was subsiding. One day about a week in, I woke up feeling light, like my depression had lifted. Then I realized that I hadn't eaten since 4 pm the day before. I was distracted and forgot supper. I guess that happens, but it showed me that I don't need three meals a day, as they say. If I didn't have so much protein in my body from dinner, maybe my body could not spare so much for autoimmune processes. Or maybe if my organs were resting and not moving so much with digestion, so they did not make so many extra movements and enzymes. Maybe my body was getting rid of toxins. Perhaps this approach was the secret to getting well from my RA. So now I do IF, and I restrict my solid food, but I drink all the water I want. Over three months, my condition has improved a lot; I'm a lot more flexible, and I have no more reflux esophagitis!

The only bad thing is that I have to stick with this for life. I broke my regimen once, and my symptoms flared up like clockwork. This plan will be for life. But it's not so bad. It is super easy to follow. The elders knew something when they said not to eat after 6!"

Jane's Fasting Story

"A bit about me. I hit 210 pounds (I'm 5'6" and 28, so yeah, I was obese), and I hated looking at myself in photos or the mirror. I was humiliated by the scale in the doctor's office. I knew that it was time to do something. I tried a bunch of diets—even keto. I couldn't follow them long enough to see long-term results. My friend said I was losing mostly water weight. I decided to try IF at her suggestion, fasting 16/8. So, I eat between 9 and 5, and then I don't eat from 5 to 9. This schedule works since I go to work at 10 so I can grab breakfast and feel fulfilled as I work.

The weight loss has been slow but sure—definitely a minus for IF but it's still weight loss and it's healthier than starving yourself. I believe you should lose no more than 10 pounds per month, and that's what I've been doing. I'm glad I tried this approach, and I recommend it to anyone."

Melissa's Fasting Story

"IF was perfect for me, since I have problems with breakfast. I chose to eat from 12-8 and not eat from 8-12. I barely notice that I'm fasting since I'm mostly asleep then. I have lost 7 pounds in a month, just sleeping when I don't eat. It's terrifically easy. No diet to follow, either.

The only minus is that sometimes I can't meet my caloric intake. I just don't have time. I am using Fat Secret and trying to meet my quota."

Candace's Fasting Story

"I was fifty pounds overweight, and then I got the worst news: My cholesterol was high, and my fasting blood sugar was 190. The doctor said I was in pre-diabetes. I was only 32! And I had a little boy at home to worry about. The idea of losing everything due to diabetes scared me, so I knew I needed to change. I looked into diets ideal for prediabetics, and something about intermittent fasting came up. I looked into it more and decided to start.

No lie, it was not easy. I am used to getting up throughout the night to snack. My favorite hobby is relaxing at home with my husband and eating lots of snacks, too. And we love to go out and eat whenever we're hungry. I had to learn a lot of discipline and control. I started by not eating for 16 hours and didn't think I could do it. I tried eating a teaspoon of almond butter and drinking water when I felt hungry, and that really helped.

Well, now I'm eight pounds away from my goal weight, meaning I've lost 42 pounds in the past six months. My cholesterol is better, and my doctor says I am no longer pre-diabetic. Plus, I feel better. Our sex life is so much better. He has lost weight doing this plan with me, too, and we are so happy."

CHAPTER 33:

Stay Motivated for the Fast

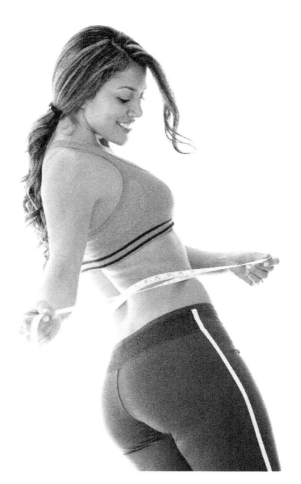

Do you know what a fasting regime and New Year resolutions have in common? They start great for a couple of months. First going to the second month; doing well. The third month; some hitches here and there. By the 6th or 7th month, some people have a problem remembering what their resolutions were in the first place. In this case, some will not remember their proposed fasting plans.

If you have fallen by the wayside, you'll be relieved to know you're not alone. Even the most enthusiastic fitness guru struggles with staying on course. If you have already missed a few steps, you can start all over again and get it right this time.

Sample these tips which will help you stay motivated:

1. Get an Accountability Partner

Having someone alongside you with similar goals can keep you on course. With the internet, your accountability partner can even be in another continent. The point here is that you're answerable to someone. You know what being answerable does to you? It makes you do things even when you don't feel like it. Like when you don't feel like getting up and going to work, but you remember you have a boss to answer to, and you jump out of bed. The accountability partner for your fasting journey may be your peer, but questions will still be asked.

This also comes with a level of competition. If your partner can fast for 24 hours, or manage on a certain number of calories, why can't you? And who lost more pounds this week? You don't want to be the one trailing, at least not every time. This accountability/competition relationship will ensure that you stay on track when you have otherwise fallen off the radar.

It is possible to achieve more with an accountability partner as opposed to a mentor. A mentor strikes an imposing figure, sort of talking down at you from a high horse. Accountability partners are at your level, demanding of you the much they demand of themselves.

2. Keep Informed

How much do you know about intermittent fasting? The more you know, the easier it will be for you to go through the process. Read blogs and watch videos to see what other women, and indeed men have to say about the fast. You'll realize that you're not alone in the issues you're experiencing.

This will also help you keep your expectations realistic. When it comes to weight loss, women can be impatient. A few days on a diet and you're already in front of the mirror looking for changes. Don't worry; we've all been there!

You know by now that intermittent fasting is a way to lose weight fast; but how fast is fast? Getting the right information from those who have gone through the fast will let you know what to expect, and you'll be better prepared to deal with the process.

3. Set Goals with Rewards

Setting milestones with some goodies attached to them will keep you going even when your body and mind tell you otherwise. Keep in mind that the reward, in this case, is not food-related.

Why can't you treat your sweet tooth as a reward? Well, to begin with, what you'd be saying to your mind is that the healthy foods you're eating are a punishment of sort, and only after eating them will you get some 'good' food. Secondly, if you indulge in sugary and fatty treats, you'll only roll back on the gains already made. We don't want any of that, do we?

Your goal here is mainly weight loss, among other health gains. Once you've reached a goal of losing a certain number of pounds in a set time, you can treat yourself to a shopping trip for new clothes. Enjoy fitting in clothes that you would not have worn previously. As you look at yourself in the mirror and admire the new you, you'll be even more motivated to work towards your next goal.

4. Concentrate on Positive Feelings

How do you feel after shedding some pounds? I'm sure you're enjoying fitting into a smaller size of outfits, looking more presentable, feeling confident, being physically active without straining, and so on.

Let these feelings color your day. Every time a thought crops upon how hungry you are, or how many foods you can no longer eat, remind yourself how dashing you look in that new dress. If you catch yourself staring at the clock gloomily counting how many more hours you have left on your fast, remind yourself that you can now make work presentations more confidently, presenting a positive body image.

Every time a negative feeling lingers, counter it with a positive thought and watch your energy revive.

5. Healthy-Eating Mind

Reprogram your mind to look at intermittent fasting, and indeed healthy eating as a whole as a positive lifestyle and not retribution. We're so accustomed to this random lifestyle where we eat what we want when we want it; that anything short of that feels like a punishment. Living healthy is choosing to be kind to your body, and knowing that it will remit the kindness right back. Think of your body for a moment as a separate entity from yourself. How would it feel when constantly being fed the wrong foods that bring you terrible effects? How would it feel to constantly be fed on too much food and you have to strain to digest? If your body could speak, it could possibly ask these questions.

Feed it on the right foods, because it is the right thing to do. Give it just the right amount, without overloading it with unnecessary carbs, sugar, and fats. And give it a break from all the digesting work occasionally, who does not like a good rest?

6. Visualize the Future

Just picture how your future will turn out if you keep living this healthy lifestyle. You'll be disease-free, active, radiant, and energetic. You'll improve your longevity, enjoying a longer, fuller life.

What's the other side of the coin? A life is ridden with disease. I'm sure you know such people, maybe even in your family, whose lives have been dimmed by disease. They're no longer able to do the things they enjoy. Their activity level is largely reduced if not cut off altogether. They are dependent on others to assist them even with minor roles. They carry medicine wherever they go. Isn't the idea of such a life horrifying, especially in a case where different choices were all was needed for a different turnout?

Choosing health is choosing life. If you still have the chance, this is an opportunity that you have to embrace. You work so hard to ensure your later days will see you age gracefully, do not let unhealthy living take this dream away from you.

7. Join a Community of Like Minds

Thank God for the internet; we can now form groups with people of similar interests even from different continents. Search the internet for women in intermittent fasting, and you should be able to find such groups. You can then exchange messages, photos, and videos of your progress. With a group also comes competition. We agree our bodies are different, but you don't want to be the one trailing the lot by losing the least weight. That only helps you stay consistent. Share experiences, tips, goals, recipes, survival tactics, and so on. Alone you can get discouraged and quit, but such a 'healthy living family' will not let you fall by the wayside.

Conclusion

Most of these female participants reported feeling more energetic and experienced better mental clarity. The women also said they were less hungry and impatient after fasting, with a greater ability to go about their day without constant snacking.

The research shows us that intermittent fasting is a great way to keep your body lean, healthy, and fit throughout menopause (and beyond)! If you're at the age where you need to make some tweaks to stay happy, healthy, and strong then we hope this article has given you some ideas!

In a Western society as fertility rates decline there is an increasing concern that more women will be diagnosed with conditions such as endometriosis. Endometriosis is a common disorder involving the growth of uterine tissue outside of the uterus. This growth can cause pelvic pain and irregular menstruation. Several studies have indicated that intermittent fasting has shown an ability to improve endometriosis, but the underlying mechanism for how it works is not fully known yet. One proposed theory is that intermittent fasting reduces your levels of estrogen, and thereby helps reduce inflammation associated with endometriosis. Currently, there are two proposed theories about how this process works and both involve intermittent fasting reducing your levels of estrogen:

1) It reduces the ability of estrogen to bind to endometrial cells (by reducing circulating estrogen).

2) It reduces the amounts of estrogen which are produced in your body and therefore your levels decrease.

Either way, this process can lead to fewer endometrial cells being formed and/or more endometrial cells being killed off. With less formation of cells, the endometriosis can become less severe, and the disease can be more effectively treated. These effects of intermittent fasting may also be related to other conditions such as diabetes which is also associated with estrogen sensitivity. Intermittent fasting could potentially help reduce calluses and other symptoms that may occur in a condition like endometriosis by helping you manage your blood sugar levels better through better insulin sensitivity.

Intermittent fasting has been shown to increase the levels of two hormones that are known to help protect brain health and improve memory. These are BDNF (Brain-derived neurotrophic factor) and HGH (Human Growth Hormone). The growth hormone also works on improving muscle mass, which can aid your body in weight loss. When it comes to BDNF, this hormone is related to the production of neurons in your brain. It helps support their survival and it also helps promote their development. Research shows that people who exercise regularly tend to have higher levels of this factor because exercise increases the amount of BDNF which is released from nerve cells.

Research suggests that BDNF may be involved in a wide range of neurodegenerative diseases such as Alzheimer's disease, Parkinson's disease, and stroke. Increasing levels of BDNF may therefore provide some degree of protection against age-related brain decline as well as other symptoms associated with neurodegenerative conditions including memory loss and impaired cognitive function. Exercise has been shown to boost BDNF levels by about 30%, which is why regular exercise generally leads to improved memory and learning ability. BDNF has also been shown to be released in response to physical activity such as weight-bearing exercise.

"One of the most important cells in your body is the neuron. A neuron is a cell that transmits information from one part of the body to another, usually the brain and spinal cord. A neuron has many nerve fibers extending out from it called dendrites, which let it connect with other neurons so it can 'talk' to them. The end of an individual nerve fiber coming out from the side of a neuron is called an axon. Axons can branch off into smaller axon terminals (axon terminals with many branches). An axon terminal may connect to the dendrites of another neuron, allowing the axon to send messages into that other neuron. If the axon terminal is sending a message into a neuron, we call it an efferent connection; if it is sending a message out from a neuron, we call it an afferent connection. Some neurons have both types of connections." - National Institutes of Health